Clinical Examination in Rheumatology

Michael Doherty MA, MD, FRCP, ILTM
Academic Rheumatology,
City Hospital, Nottingham

John Doherty BA, Dip AD
Port Hope, Ontario, Canada

ISBN 07234 1685 0

Contents

Dedication

TO EMMA, JILL, NICOLA, TARA,
DEBBIE AND SALLY

Preface

Rheumatological problems are exceedingly common in clinical practice. Although many such problems are confined to locomotor structures, the frequent combined involvement of locomotor and other systems in disease requires all doctors to have a certain basic level of rheumatological examination expertise.

The history and physical examination together provide most, if not all, the information required for the diagnosis and management of patients with rheumatological problems. Clinical examination skills are, therefore, of paramount importance. Surprisingly, however, few student rheumatology books sufficiently emphasise these skills or give clear instruction on how to perform regional examination.

This book fills that gap. It largely reflects the teaching given to fifth year clinical students at Nottingham University, and arose from the requests of these students for a written record of the clinical skills programme. Such a major emphasis on clinical skills is in keeping with the current philosophy on medical education. Other aspects of rheumatology (the rational approach to diagnosis, investigations, details of specific conditions, and management) are to be included in a planned accompanying volume, *Rheumatology - Diagnosis, Investigation, Management.*

In the Introduction a brief clarification of joint structure and classification is followed by consideration of general aspects of the history and examination. Chapter 2 describes the 'minimal' or preliminary rheumatological screen required to detect and approximately localize problems in this system. It is sufficiently brief to be easily incorporated into the standard medical systems enquiry. Subsequent chapters give more detailed information (basic anatomy, pain patterns, methods of clinical examination) to enable the determination of articular and periarticular problems at individual regions.

Throughout we have used plentiful illustrations. No book is totally comprehensive, but this volume contains sufficient information for the medical student, non-rheumatologist doctor, and allied health professionals to apply basic anatomy to recognize common and important causes of regional locomotor pain.

MICHAEL DOHERTY

1   Introduction

The locomotor system is concerned with *controlled motion*, and the structure of its integral parts reflects this functional requirement.

DEVELOPMENT AND BASIC STRUCTURE OF JOINTS

Bone, cartilage, and muscle develop from mesenchymal tissue. Their basic organisation is self-differentiating and occurs during the embryonic period (4–8 weeks). The remainder of gestation (the foetal period) is largely concerned with growth: during this period and throughout life, locomotor development is strongly influenced by movement, usage, and physical stresses, which thus help adapt locomotor tissues to their functional demands. Points worthy of note (particularly in respect of congenital skeletal anomalies) include:

- Axial development occurs in a cranial–caudal manner.
- Limb buds grow peripherally.
- Upper limbs develop a little in advance of lower limbs (insults during the period of limb development affect the distal parts of the arms more than the legs).
- The number of rays increases distally (one in the upper arm and thigh, two in the forearm and shin, three in the carpus and tarsus, five in the hand and foot).
- Dermatomes, myotomes, and sclerotomes (tissues sharing the same segmental innervation) give rise, respectively, to skin, muscle, and joint/bone tissues.

Joints are discontinuities in the skeleton that permit controlled mobility. If very little movement is required the bone-ends are firmly joined in a continuous fashion (*synarthrosis*, **1–3**), being bridged by either one of:

- Fibrous tissue (*syndesmosis*), permitting almost no motion (e.g. skull sutures).
- Cartilage (*synchondrosis*), permitting limited movement. Primary cartilaginous joints, e.g. between the epiphysis and diaphysis, are linked by hyaline cartilage, which eventually ossifies: secondary cartilaginous joints (symphyses) are joined by compressible fibrocartilage and are predominantly axial, e.g. symphysis pubis, intervertebral joints, and manubriosternal joints.

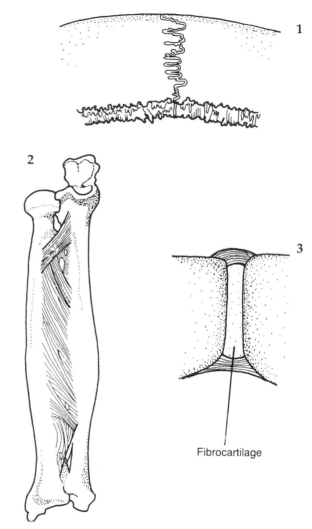

Fibrocartilage

1–3   Examples of synarthroses: (**1**) skull suture (syndesmosis); (**2**) interosseous membrane (syndesmosis); (**3**) symphysis (synchondrosis).

If a moderate or wide range of movement is required, a space develops, forming a discontinuous *diarthrosis* or *synovial joint* (**4**). In such joints, the bone-ends are covered by hyaline cartilage: in some, additional fibrocartilage pads divide the cavity completely (discs) or partially (menisci).

A **capsule** encircles the joint: its outer portion is fibrous, its inner lining forms the villous **synovial membrane**. The major functions of the latter include:

- Secretion of viscous **synovial fluid** (a modified ultrafiltrate) that fills the joint 'space', being important in lubrication and nutrition of cartilage.
- Provision of an efficient macrophage system to remove particulate and foreign matter.

The synovium possesses inward-facing fat-containing processes (plicae). **Ligaments** insert between the bones as thickened portions of capsule or as separate structures. The site of firm attachment of fibrous structures (tendon, ligament, capsule) into periosteum and bone is called the **enthesis**.

Bursae are fluid-filled sacs that facilitate smooth movement between articulating structures. Their lining lacks a basement membrane and appears identical to the synovium. **Subcutaneous bursae** (e.g. olecranon, prepatellar bursae) form after birth in response to normal external friction: **deep bursae** (e.g. subacromial bursae) usually form before birth in response to internal movement between muscles and bones, and may or may not communicate with joint cavities. **'Adventitious' bursae** (e.g. over the first metatarsal head) form in response to abnormal shearing stresses.

Muscles acting over the joint move it through its normal range — forceful movement in one direction being controlled by relaxation of antagonist muscles. The balanced action of muscles *constrains* as well as *powers* joint movement. **Tendons** anchor muscle to bone. Muscle is not required for tendon differentiation, but without good muscle strength sustained development of tendons fails. Many tendons, particularly those with a large range of motion, have sheaths (**tenosynovium**) resembling the capsule/synovium of joints to permit easy gliding movement.

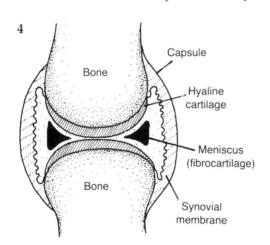

4

4 Diagrammatic structure of a synovial joint (diarthrosis).

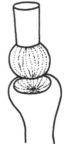

7

Pivot, swing (e.g. distal radioulnar)

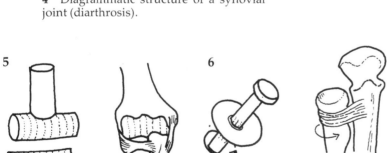

6

Pivot, peg-in-a-hole (e.g. proximal radioulnar)

5

Hinge (e.g. humeroulnar)

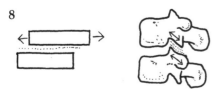

8

Sliding (e.g. intervertebral apophyseal)

9

Ball and socket (e.g. glenohumeral).

5–9 Joint classification according to movement.

The range of movement and stability of individual synovial joints varies according to:

- The shape of the articular surfaces.
- Capsular strength.
- Ligaments.
- Muscles acting across the joint.
- The presence of adjacent structures.

Descriptive classification, especially of synovial joints, is often based on the type of movement undertaken (5–9).

PRINCIPLES OF THE EXAMINATION OF A PATIENT WITH RHEUMATIC DISEASE

The rheumatological examination is an exercise in applied anatomy, with utilisation of simple provocation or stress tests. Screening of the locomotor system should be included in any full general medical examination: many rheumatic diseases involve other systems and, conversely, many 'general medical' conditions (particularly endocrine, metabolic, and neoplastic) affect locomotor structures. In this introduction, only important aspects of the locomotor history and examination will be emphasised: an accompanying systems enquiry and examination is assumed, and only aspects relating to key extra-articular target sites will be emphasised.

TERMINOLOGY

The following glossary relates to the site and nature of rheumatological problems:

Arthralgia. Pain that arises in joints (not necessarily with obvious abnormality).
Arthritis/Arthropathy. Objective joint abnormality.
Chondropathy. A process that results in loss of cartilage.
Monoarthritis. Arthropathy of only one joint.
Oligoarthritis/Pauciarticular disease. Arthritis that affects from two to four joints (or small joint groups, e.g. 'wrist').
Polyarthritis. Arthritis that affects more than four joints (or groups).
Synovitis. Clinically apparent synovial joint inflammation.
Capsulitis. Inflammation/disease of capsule.
Tenosynovitis. Tendon sheath inflammation.
Tendinitis. Inflammation of tendon.
Bursitis. Inflammation of a bursa.
Enthesopathy. Inflammation/abnormality of an enthesis.

Myopathy. Disease/abnormality of muscle.
Myositis. Inflammatory disease of muscle.
Subluxation. Where two articular surfaces are abnormally aligned but remain in direct contact.
Dislocation. Where two articular surfaces are so out of alignment that there is no direct surface-to-surface contact.

SYMPTOMS

Locomotor symptoms that require clear delineation in the history are summarised in **10**. It is important to ascertain:

- The site/distribution of involvement.
- Chronological onset.
- Preceding provoking factors.
- Factors which worsen or improve symptoms.
- Symptom response to health interventions.

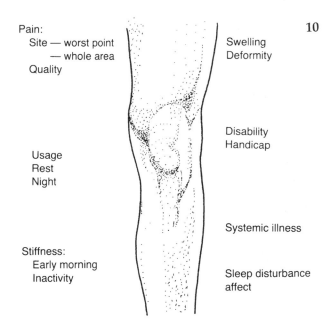

Pain:
Site — worst point
— whole area
Quality

Swelling
Deformity

Disability
Handicap

Usage
Rest
Night

Systemic illness

Stiffness:
Early morning
Inactivity

Sleep disturbance
affect

10

10 Important locomotor symptoms.

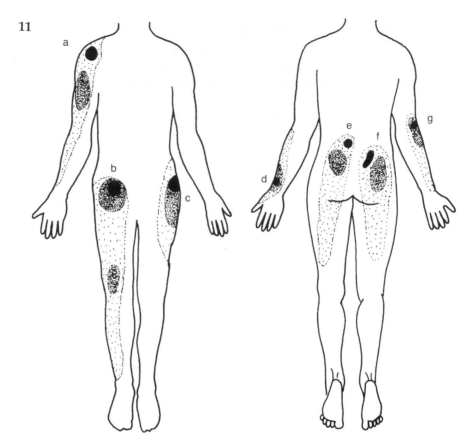

11 Examples of pain radiation from articular and periarticular sites: (a) gleno-humeral joint/rotator cuff; (b) hip joint; (c) trochanteric bursitis; (d) de Quervain's tenosynovitis; (e) lumbar facet joint syndrome; (f) sacroiliac joint; (g) tennis elbow syndrome.

Pain

This is the usual, most important symptom for the patient. The examiner must be certain of the site of pain. Patient terminology (e.g. 'shoulder' or 'hip') may be misleading; the patient should point to the site of maximum intensity and map out the area over which pain is experienced.

Articular or periarticular pain may radiate widely and present distant from the originating structure (**11**). Such **'referred'** pain is an error in perception at the sensory cortex, reflecting shared innervation by structures derived from the same embryonic segment (which divides into dermatome, myotome, and sclerotome). Cortical cells most commonly receive stimuli from skin: when the same cells receive, for the first time, a painful stimulus from a deeply situated myotomal/sclerotomal structure they interpret the signal on past experience and 'feel' pain in the area of skin (dermatome) which shares that connection. An important difference is that the pain is felt deeply, rather than in the skin itself, and its boundaries are indistinct. In general:

- Referred pain radiates segmentally without crossing the midline.
- The dermatome often extends more distally than the myotome, so pain is mainly referred distally. The more distal the originating structure the more accurate the pain localisation is likely to be.
- In addition to pain referral, tenderness may also be experienced at a distant site.
- Dermatomes are variable between individuals — the precise area of pain referral may thus differ between patients with the same loco-motor problem.

- In general, the more superficial a soft-tissue structure the more precise its pain localisation (pain from deep, but hard, structures, such as bone and periosteum, hardly radiates at all).
- Massage over the area of referred pain may improve rather than worsen the pain (whereas pressure over the originating structure may reproduce the pain).

Quality of pain is generally unhelpful. Exceptions include (1) sharp, shooting pain that travels a distance, characteristic of root entrapment, and (2) extreme pain ('worst experienced'), typical of crystal synovitis. Although topographical localisation is at the sensory cortex level, pain appreciation and severity is determined by cells in the supra-orbital region of the frontal lobes, which explains why the patient's emotional state has such an influence over 'severity'. The memory of pain is retained in the temporal lobes: duration rather than severity determines recall.

Factors that exacerbate or ameliorate the pain should be sought. Pain confined to **usage** suggests a mechanical problem, particularly if it worsens during use and quickly improves on resting. **Rest pain** and pain worse at the beginning rather than end of usage implies a marked inflammatory component. **Night pain** is a distressing symptom: it reflects intra-osseous hypertension and accompanies serious problems such as avascular necrosis or bone collapse adjacent to a severely arthritic joint. Persistent (day and night) **'bony pain'** is characteristic of neoplastic invasion.

Stiffness

Stiffness is a subjective sensation of resistance to movement ('tightness') that probably reflects fluid distension of the limiting boundary of the inflamed tissue (capsule, tenosynovium, bursa). It is most marked on arising from bed, and following inactivity or rest. As normal usage resumes, fluid clearance from the inflamed structure is encouraged and stiffness 'wears off'. Duration and severity of **early morning** and **inactivity stiffness** thus reflect the degree of local inflammation.

Swelling/deformity

Patients may notice swelling, discoloration, or abnormal contour or alignment of a locomotor structure. Although 'deformity' describes any abnormality, the term is usually restricted to malalignment or subluxation/dislocation.

Disability and handicap

Disability is present when a tissue, organ, or system cannot function adequately. **Handicap** is when disability interferes with daily activities or social/occupational performance. Marked disability need not necessarily cause handicap (e.g. an above-knee amputee may not be disadvantaged in a sedentary job); conversely, minor disability may produce major handicap (e.g. an ingrowing toenail in a professional footballer). Therefore, both require separate assessment.

Systemic illness

Inflammatory locomotor disease ($\pm$ multisystem involvement) may trigger a marked acute phase response and cause non-specific symptoms of systemic upset; for example, fevers (particularly at night), reduced appetite, weight loss, fatigability, lethargy, and irritability. The patient may volunteer no specific complaints but just feel 'ill'. In the elderly, particularly, florid acute inflammation (e.g. crystal synovitis) may cause confusion.

Sleep disturbance/affect

Several factors may interfere with normal sleep patterns and associate with anxiety and depression. For example:

- Chronic pain.
- Triggering of the acute phase response.
- Reasonable anxiety concerning deformity and morbidity.
- CNS side-effects from pain-relieving drugs.
- Severe arthropathy (hip, knee especially) may compromise sexual function, and contribute to marital/social disharmony.

Features of masked or overt depression (e.g. psychomotor retardation, constipation, weepiness, no thoughts of the future) should specifically be sought, particularly in those with severe locomotor disease. Poor sleep pattern is also a feature of fibromyalgia.

SIGNS

Principal headings for signs at any region are shown in **12**. The order of examination applicable to most regions is (1) **inspection at rest**, (2) **inspection during movement**, and (3) **palpation (often with movement)**.

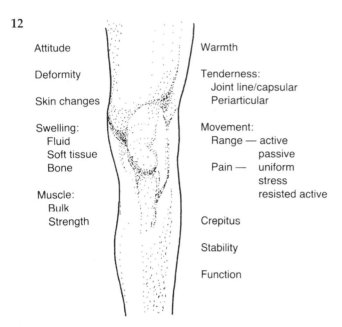

Attitude

Deformity

Skin changes

Swelling:
  Fluid
  Soft tissue
  Bone

Muscle:
  Bulk
  Strength

Warmth

Tenderness:
  Joint line/capsular
  Periarticular

Movement:
  Range — active
            passive
  Pain — uniform
            stress
            resisted active

Crepitus

Stability

Function

12 Important locomotor signs.

Attitude

Observe the way the patient positions an affected region. A joint with synovitis has intra-articular hypertension and is most comfortable in the position that minimises pressure increase. Such a position (generally mild–mid flexion) is mainly determined by the configuration of the capsule. For example, glenohumeral synovitis is most comfortable with the arm adducted and internally rotated as if in a sling; conversely, the opposite movements, abduction and external rotation, are the earliest affected and most uncomfortable since these maximise intra-articular hypertension. The attitude and pattern of restricted movement may thus suggest the underlying problem.

Deformity

Although deformities may be observed at rest, most become more apparent on weight bearing or usage. It should be determined whether the deformity is correctable (usually implying soft-tissue factors in causation) or non-correctable (usually capsular restriction or joint damage). Many conditions associate with characteristic deformities (e.g. at the knee, **13–17**), but no deformity is pathognomonic of one disease. Short-hand terms are used for combined deformities (e.g. 'swan-neck' finger deformity for hyperextension at the proximal and fixed flexion at the distal interphalangeal joint).

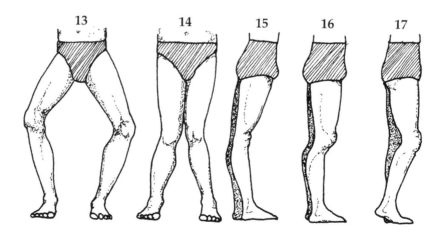

13–17 Principal knee deformities: (**13**) varus: typical of osteoarthritis (a focal condition maximally affecting the medial compartment); (**14**) valgus: typical of pan-compartmental inflammatory conditions, e.g. rheumatoid and psoriatic arthritis, pyrophosphate arthropathy; (**15**) recurvatum: common in generalised hypermobility; (**16**) posterior tibial subluxation: characteristic of arthropathies occurring during growth, e.g. haemophilia, juvenile chronic arthropathy; (**17**) fixed flexion: common in various arthropathies.

Skin changes

Overlying scars or skin disease (e.g. psoriasis) may be important clues to causation. **Erythema** (commonly followed by desquamation) is an important sign reflecting periarticular inflammation: although this may occur in several conditions (*Table 1*), a red joint or bursa should always raise suspicion of sepsis or crystals.

Swelling

This may be due to fluid, soft tissue, or bone. Fluid within a joint collects initially and maximally at sites of least resistance within the capsular confines, producing characteristic swelling at individual sites (**18–20**); for example:

- Knee effusions fill the medial dimple and, subsequently, the suprapatellar pouch, giving a horseshoe swelling above and around the patella.
- Interphalangeal joint synovitis is initially apparent as posterolateral swelling between the extensor tendon and lateral collateral ligaments.
- Glenohumeral effusion fills the triangular depression between the clavicle and the deltoid, in front of pectoralis.
- Ankle effusions present anteriorly.

Table 1.   Causes of erythema overlying joints.

Major
   Sepsis
   Crystals (gout, pseudogout, calcific periarthritis)

Minor
   Palindromic rheumatism
   Acute Reiter's or reactive arthropathy
   Early Heberden's or Bouchard's nodes
   Inflammatory (erosive) osteoarthritis (hands)
   Erythema nodosum arthropathy
   Rheumatic fever

Erythema implies periarticular inflammation

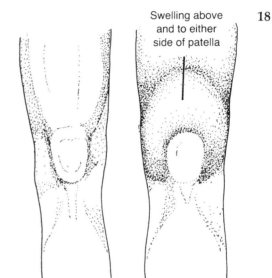

Swelling above and to either side of patella   **18**

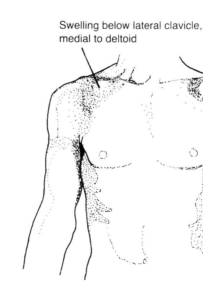

19   Posterolateral swelling Tightness/loss of skin creases

Swelling below lateral clavicle, medial to deltoid   **20**

18–20   Characteristic swellings produced by synovial hypertrophy/effusion: (**18**) the knee; (**19**) finger interphalangeal joint; (**20**) shoulder.

For small fluid volumes in a confined cavity, a **bulge sign** may be produced (e.g. at the knee, massage fluid from the medial dimple to the lateral aspect of the patella and back again). Larger volumes produce a **balloon sign** (fluctuance), where pressure over one point causes 'ballooning' at other parts of the swelling (**21**). This is the most specific sign for fluid (joints, bursae). **Capsular swelling** is the most specific sign of synovitis: swelling is delineated by the capsular confines and becomes firmer towards the extremes of movement (palpate during passive movement).

Tenderness

Precise localisation of tenderness is perhaps the most useful sign in determining the cause of the patient's problem (**22, 23**). **Joint-line/capsular tenderness** is localised to the joint boundary and signifies arthropathy/capsular disease if present around the whole margin (localised joint-line tenderness suggests localised intracapsular pathology, e.g. anterior medial tibiofemoral compartment tenderness with medial meniscal tears). **Periarticular point tenderness** away from the joint line usually signifies bursitis or enthesopathy.

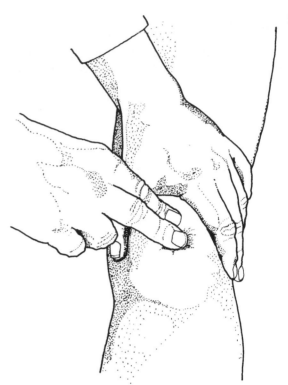

21 'Balloon sign' at knee. Pressure over patella with one hand causes 'ballooning' of the other hand closely applied over suprapatellar expansion.

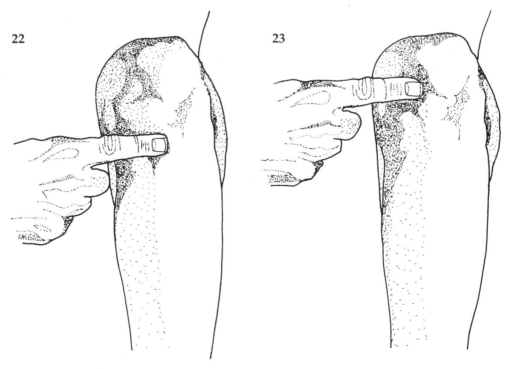

22, 23 Example of differentiation between periarticular and joint-line tenderness at the knee: (**22**) tenderness confined to patella tendon insertion into the tibial tubercle (Osgood–Schlatter disease); (**23**) tenderness confined to anterior joint line of medial tibiofemoral compartment (medial meniscal injury).

Muscle

Muscle wasting is a common sign, but can be difficult to detect — particularly in the elderly. Synovitis quickly produces local spinal reflex inhibition of muscles acting across the joint: wasting can be rapid (within several days in septic arthritis). Severe arthropathy produces widespread periarticular wasting: localised wasting is more characteristic of a mechanical tendon/muscle problem or nerve entrapment. Power is more important than bulk and can be tested either by grading from 0–5 (*Table 2*: appropriate, for example, for proximal girdle and neck muscle weakness in polymyositis), or by assessment of functional capabilities (more appropriate, for example, for weakness of small hand muscles in rheumatoid arthritis).

Table 2. Muscle power grading (Medical Research Council scale).

Grade No.	Definition
0	No visible contraction
1	Visible or palpable contraction without motion
2	Motion only with gravity eliminated
3	Motion against gravity
4	Motion against gravity and an applied load
5	Normal power, i.e. against a significant load

Warmth

This is one of the cardinal signs of inflammation. The back of the hand is a sensitive thermometer for comparing skin temperature above, over, and below an inflamed structure.

Movement

Assess range of active and passive movement, with comparison between sides (to demonstrate unilateral reduction). Synovitis reduces most or all joint movements (**'proportional' limitation or 'capsular pattern'**), though some are affected initially and maximally, e.g. external rotation and abduction at the glenohumeral joint. Tenosynovitis and periarticular lesions affect movement in one plane only. Synovitis and arthropathy cause similar reduction of active and passive movement: far greater passive than active movement suggests a muscle/tendon/motor problem.

The pattern of pain on movement is of diagnostic significance. Pain absent or minimal in the mid-range but increasing towards the extremes of restricted movement is 'stress pain'. **Universal stress pain** (in most/all directions) is the most sensitive sign of synovitis (**24**). **Selective stress pain** (in one plane of movement only) is characteristic of a localised intra- or periarticular lesion. Pain uniformly present throughout a range of movement usually reflects mechanical rather than inflammatory problems (*Table 3*).

Ranges of movement are age-, sex- and race-dependent. Attempts to measure degrees of movement (by a variety of instruments) are inaccurate, have poor reproducibility, and are not recommended for routine examination purposes.

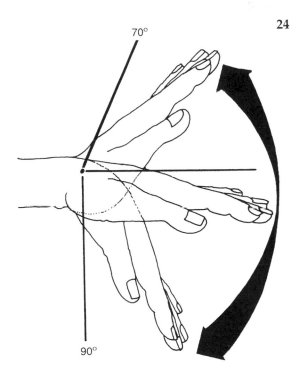

24

70°

90°

24 Stress pain at the wrist: no discomfort in mild flexion, but progressive pain towards the extremes of restricted flexion and extension.

Table 3. Summary of principal signs relating to synovitis, tenosynovitis, and joint damage.

Synovitis
    Held in neutral
    Decreased movement *ALL* planes
    Stress pain *ALL* directions
    CAPSULAR swelling/effusion
    JOINT-LINE/CAPSULAR tenderness
    Increased warmth
    ± Fine crepitus

    CAPSULAR SWELLING is the most specific sign
    STRESS PAIN is the most sensitive sign

Tenosynovitis
    Joint positioned to decrease tension
    Decreased movement in plane of tendon
    SELECTIVE stress pain
    Linear swelling
    Localised (linear) tenderness
    ± Fine crepitus
    ± Triggering

Joint damage
    Abnormal shape/subluxation
    Coarse crepitus
    Decreased movement
    ± Ligamentous stress pain/instability
    ± Synovitis

A useful method for demonstrating periarticular problems is **'resisted active (isometric) movement'** (**25–27**). The patient pushes against the examiner's restraining hand, to contract the muscle of interest without moving adjacent joints. If the patient's

25–27 Resisted active movement and stress tests: (**25**) attempted external rotation at the shoulder causes upper arm pain in an infraspinatus/teres minor rotator cuff lesion; (**26**) resisted wrist extension reproduces lateral epicondyle pain in tennis elbow; (**27**) Finkelstein's test: passive ulnar flexion with thumb held stretches abductor pollicis longus and extensor pollicis brevis to reproduce the pain of de Quervain's tenosynovitis.

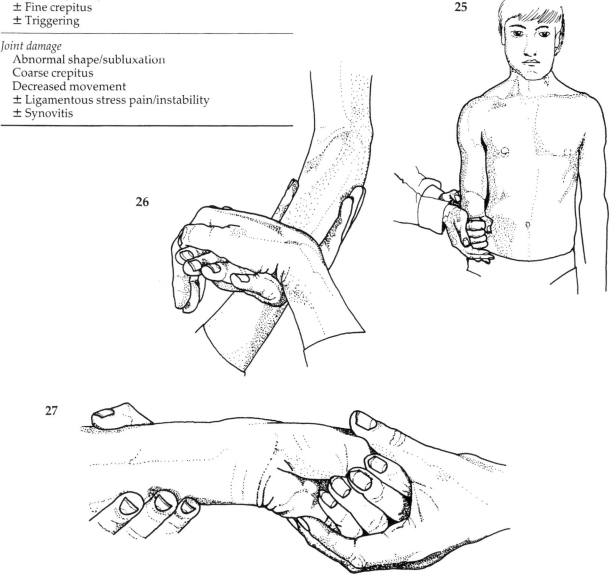

pain is reproduced (and no joint has moved) it probably arises from muscle, tendon, or tendon insertion. For example, resisted hip adduction produces medial groin pain in adductor tendonitis; resisted glenohumeral abduction produces upper-arm pain with supraspinatus muscle/tendon lesions; resisted wrist extension reproduces lateral epicondyle pain in tennis elbow. Similarly, passive **stress tests** reproduce pain by stretching the responsible ligament/tendon (e.g. Finkelstein's test for de Quervain's tenosynovitis, where passive stretch of the abductor pollicis longus and extensor pollicis brevis muscles reproduces pain).

Crepitus

Crepitus is palpable crunching that is present throughout the movement of the involved structure. **Fine crepitus** may be audible by stethoscope and is not transmitted through adjacent bone: it may accompany inflammation of tendon sheath, bursa, or synovium. **Coarse crepitus** may be audible at a distance and is palpable through bone: it usually reflects cartilage or bone damage. Other noises include **ligamentous snaps** (usually single, loud, painless: common around the upper femur as 'clicking hips'); **'cracking'** by joint distraction (common at finger joints and caused by production of an intra-articular gas bubble — 'cracking' cannot be repeated until the bubble has resorbed); and reproducible **clonking** noises at irregular surfaces (e.g. the scapula moving on the ribs).

Stability

Localised ligamentous or capsular instability may result from traumatic or inflammatory lesions. Arthropathy (particularly inflammatory) may produce instability via cartilage loss and capsular inflammation, as well as by ligamentous rupture. Stability is determined by demonstration of excessive movement on stressing the joint. Comparison with the other side is often helpful.

Function

Function is assessed by observation during normal usage (e.g. rising from a chair and walking for hips, knees and feet; power grip and fine-precision pinch for the hand). **Activities of daily living,** or **ADL** (e.g. dressing, brushing teeth, going to the toilet unaided, and cooking) are of direct relevance to the patient, and screening questions or observations of ADL are invaluable in assessment. **Handicap** is mainly determined by questioning related to work and social activities. The World Health Organisation define *health status* as 'a comprehensive state of physical, mental and social wellbeing', emphasising that psychological and emotional factors, specific to patients rather than to their condition, are important in determining the functional impact and effects of disease on the individual. A variety of tested and validated questionnaires/scoring systems are now available for both functional and quality of life (overall health status) assessments.

Generalised hypermobility

This is one of two generalised conditions (with fibromyalgia) that is easily missed unless specifically considered.

Ten per cent of people fall within the lax end of a normal spectrum of joint mobility. Although normal, such hypermobility may contribute to locomotor problems (e.g. enthesopathy, disloca-tion). Within this 10% are also the small number of individuals with disease-related hypermobility (e.g. Marfan's syndrome, Ehlers–Danlos syndrome, acromegaly). Generalised hypermobility can be screened for by using a modified Beighton score (*Table 4*, **28**).

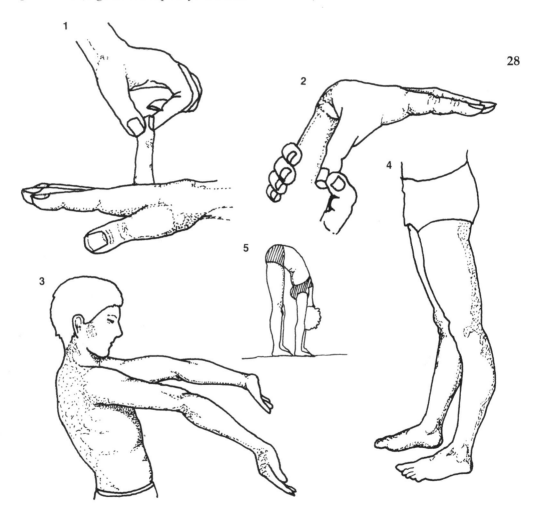

28 Features of generalised hypermobility (see *Table 4*).

Table 4. Recognition of generalised hypermobility.

1 Extend little finger >90° (1 point each side)
2 Bring thumb back parallel to/touching forearm (1 point each)
3 Extend elbow >10° (1 point each)
4 Extend knee >10° (1 point each)
5 Touch floor with flat of hand, legs straight (1 point)

Maximum score = 9
Hypermobile = 6 or more

Fibromyalgia (non-restorative sleep disorder)

This common syndrome is characterised by:

- Poor sleep pattern (waking unrefreshed).
- Fatigability, lethargy.
- Irritability.
- Multiple regional pain (predominantly axial, often 'all over'), unresponsive to analgesics.
- Hypersensitivity of normal tender sites (**29**).

Fibromyalgia may be **primary** (particularly affecting middle-aged women) or **secondary** (superimposed on a recognised painful condition). It is suggested by the features in the history and confirmed principally by the finding of hypertender sites (with no hyperalgesia at other control sites) and elimination of other causes of widespread aches and pains (e.g. hyperparathyroidism, hypothyroidism, lupus).

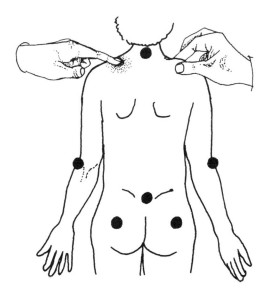

29

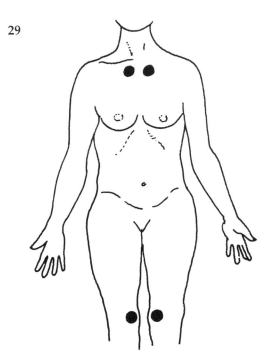

- Low cervical spine
- Mid-point of supraspinatus
- Skin roll tenderness over trapezius
- 1 cm distal to lateral epicondyle
- Low lumbar spine
- Upper gluteal area

- Pectoralis, maximum lateral to second costochondral junction
- Medial fat pad of knee

29 Common tender sites in fibromyalgia syndrome.

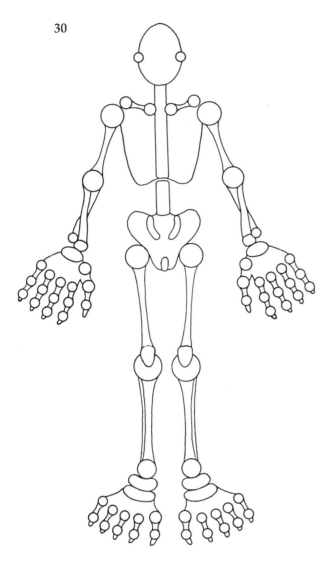

30 Homunculus for annotated recording of locomotor signs.

Table 5. Causes of nodules plus arthropathy.

Common
  Rheumatoid arthritis
  Gout (nodules = 'tophi')
  Hyperlipidaemia (nodules = 'xanthomata')

Rare
  Systemic lupus (small nodules)
  Rheumatic fever (small nodules)
  Multicentric reticulohistiocytosis
  Polyarteritis nodosa
  Sarcoidosis

Most nodules (and small vessel vasculitis) occur over extensor surfaces and pressure areas

Recording locomotor signs

Although physical findings can be written in note form, annotation around skeleton charts, or homunculi (**30**), is recommended. Such visual recording greatly aids pattern recognition.

Aspects of the general examination

In the context of a complete systems examination, particular emphasis may be given to skin (including scalp, umbilicus, and natal cleft for occult psoriasis), nails, mucous membranes (especially orogenital and nasal), and eyes.

Nodules are particularly relevant to locomotor disease (*Table 5*). Whatever their cause, nodules are usually most prominent over poorly covered extensor surfaces (e.g. back of the hands, elbow, posterior heel, and sacrum).

Nail changes of interest include clubbing (most causes of clubbing have locomotor associations, but hypertrophic pulmonary osteoarthropathy and fibrosing alveolitis are particularly relevant); 'thimble pitting', onycholysis and nail dystrophy (psoriatic arthropathy, chronic Reiter's); nailfold hyperaemia (often prominent in dermatomyositis); splinter haemorrhages (small-vessel vasculitis); and Beau's lines (systemic illness) (**31–34**). Rheumatoid is the commonest pathological cause of **palmar erythema** (above cirrhosis or thyrotoxicosis).

Mucous membrane lesions may be asymptomatic (common in Reiter's/reactive arthropathy) or symptomatic (most usual in lupus, vasculitides, Behçet's syndrome), and inspection of orogenital and nasal mucosae for ulcers and telangiectasia is warranted. Absence of saliva either side of the frenulum suggests sicca syndrome.

Eye changes (*Table 6*) include **episcleritis** and **scleritis** (rheumatoid, vasculitides, polychondritis); **iritis** (ankylosing spondylitis, chronic Reiter's); **iridocyclitis** (pauciarticular juvenile chronic arthritis); and **conjunctivitis** (acute Reiter's syndrome, sicca syndrome). Fundoscopy, in particular, may be relevant in suspected vasculitis.

31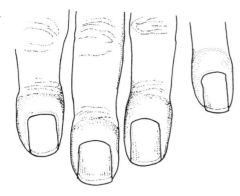

32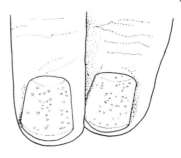

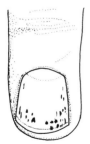

33

34

31–34 Nail changes: (31) clubbing; (32) thimble pitting; (33) onycholysis, nail dystrophy (plus distal interphalangeal joint swelling); (34) splinter haemorrhages.

Table 6. Characteristics of important causes of a red eye.

Conjunctivitis
  Itchiness, irritation
  Diffusely red due to engorged vessel network
  Redness extends over bulbar surface of eyelids
  Vessels can be moved over surface
  Mucopurulent discharge common ('sticky eye')

Episcleritis
  Usually asymptomatic
  Diffuse or localised ('nodular' episcleritis)
  Bright red flush, individual vessels often visible
  Vessels cannot be moved over eyeball
  Vessels constrict to local adrenaline drops (1:1000)

Scleritis
  Usually painful, often severe
  Deep red/purple colour, vessels indistinct
  Deep vessels do not constrict to adrenaline drops
  Often accompanied by episcleritis
  May be visual disturbance
  Localised ('nodular') scleritis causes elevated lesion due to oedema
  Diffuse scleritis causes less pain but may involve cornea, causing keratitis
    and keratolysis ('corneal melt')
  Healed scleritis may leave sclera more transparent and permit the dark
    underlying choroid to be seen ('scleromalacia')

Acute iritis
  Severe throbbing pain
  Blurring of vision, photophobia, lacrimation
  Usually involves only one eye at a time: light in other eye will exacerbate
    pain as iris constricts
  Small vessels of limbus are engorged ('ciliary flush')
  Small spastic pupil, may be irregular (due to posterior adhesions or
    'synechiae')
  Clouding of aqueous ± anterior chamber pus collection inferiorly
    ('hypopyon')

ASSIMILATION OF FINDINGS

Following the history and examination it is often helpful to organise findings under the titles in **35**. Consideration of just age and sex will narrow diagnostic possibilities considerably. For arthropathy the temporal presentation (acute, chronic, or relapsing), number of joints involved, distribution, and degree of inflammatory component (*Table 7*) will then usually suggest the most likely diagnosis with few options: the presence of particular extra-articular features may narrow possibilities further. Any investigations can then be highly selected and a rheumatologic 'screen' with multiple investigations should never be required.

Only an adequate history and examination will permit correct diagnosis and an appropriate management plan. It should be remembered that apparently mundane and localised lesions (e.g. Achilles tendinitis) may be the presenting feature of a widespread or multisystem condition.

Table 7. Symptoms and signs that might suggest a marked inflammatory component to arthropathy.

Local
Early morning stiffness
Inactivity stiffness
Swelling
Warmth
Effusion
Capsular swelling
Stress pain

Systemic
Weight loss
Fevers, sweats
Lethargy, irritability, depression
Anaemia

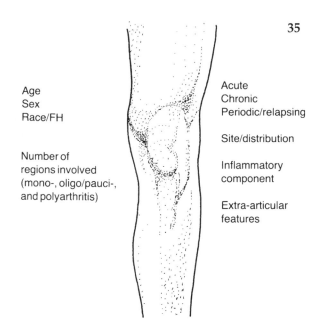

Age
Sex
Race/FH

Number of
regions involved
(mono-, oligo/pauci-,
and polyarthritis)

35

Acute
Chronic
Periodic/relapsing

Site/distribution

Inflammatory
component

Extra-articular
features

35 Principal considerations when organising findings.

2 Preliminary Rheumatological Examination

An exhaustive history and extensive examination for all conceivable rheumatological abnormalities in every patient are time-consuming and unnecessary. As with other systems, a brief screening procedure to pick up problems in defined regions is more appropriate. If an abnormality is detected, a more detailed examination of affected regions (as described in subsequent chapters) can be undertaken to define the problem more precisely.

Screening is a compromise between brevity and sensitivity to detect abnormality. To screen a joint for arthropathy the movement that is affected first and maximally is selected for scrutiny: if normal, other movements of that joint can be omitted. Many such movements have functional importance, and the screen is one of function as well as joint/muscle abnormality. Students will develop their own variation of the 'minimum screen' for the locomotor just as for other systems, and the following is offered as a guide rather than a doctrine. Such a screen can readily be included within the systems enquiry and examination that comprises the routine medical clerical procedure. Certain aspects (e.g. gait) overlap with screening of other systems (particularly neurological) and in the setting of a routine clerking procedure the screen takes only a minute or so to perform.

SCREENING HISTORY

Pain and stiffness are the most common symptoms, and functional impairment the most important consequence of rheumatological abnormality. Therefore, reasonable screening questions are:

'Have you any pain or stiffness in your muscles, joints or back?'
'Can you dress yourself completely without any difficulty?'
'Can you walk up and down stairs without any difficulty?'

Dressing is a daily event with which the patient readily identifies in terms of problems. Ability to dress completely (including shoes and socks) is a sensitive functional test of most upper and lower limb joints, and if the patient has no pain or difficulty dressing then significant or widespread locomotor disease is unlikely. If the patient can go up and down stairs without any problem then most lower limb muscles and joints are functioning well: up and down stairs is a better test of hip and knee, particularly patellofemoral, problems than walking on the flat. If none of these questions detects a problem, further questioning is unlikely to do so. If a problem is found, more detailed questioning is obviously warranted. (Note that the two functional questions are not specific to locomotor disease and may have been included elsewhere in a systems enquiry.)

SCREENING EXAMINATION

This mainly comprises *inspection at rest* and *inspection during selected movements*. Brief palpation and stress tests of joints commonly involved in inflammatory arthropathy (metacarpophalangeal and metatarsophalangeal joints and knees) completes the screen.

The normal joint should:

- *Look normal.* With advancing age the features of a joint become more visible, and muscle bulk diminishes, without necessarily signifying disease.

- *Assume a normal resting position.* Abnormal positioning of a normal joint may result from poor postural habit, neurological abnormality, or psychogenic disorder with feigning of disease. Postural abnormalities should disappear when the patient is asked to adopt the normal position and undertake normal movement. Psychogenic posturing is often odd, inconsistent, and unique to the patient.

- *Move smoothly through its range of movement.* Articular or periarticular lesions often cause jerky, guarded movement, and the patient may use trick manoeuvres to minimise disability.

The patient should be assessed during walking, while standing, and while lying on a couch. Observation of the patient getting undressed is a further useful functional screen, though some physicians prefer to spare the patient any embarrassment this may cause. The order in which the screening is performed is unimportant, and although described here as individual procedures inspection, palpation and stress tests of a region can often be undertaken simultaneously. The procedure is facilitated and hastened if the examiner undertakes the movements so that the patient can see and copy exactly what is required.

Inspection of the walking patient

With the patient barefoot and undressed to their underwear, observe their gait as they walk forwards, turn and walk back again. Scrutinise movements of arms, pelvis, hips, knees, hindfoot, midfoot, and forefoot, in turn. Normal gait (36–39) is characterised by:

- Flowing arm movement linked to movement of the opposite leg.

- Smooth, symmetrical movement of the pelvis, rotating forward with the advancing leg.
- Hip flexion at heel strike, hip extension at toe-off.
- Knee extension at heel strike, flexion during swing.
- Normal heel strike, foot pronation in mid-stance, heel rise before push-off, and ankle dorsiflexion during swing.
- Smooth turning ability.

As the patient walks and turns, look particularly for an *antalgic gait* (40) where pain or deformity causes the patient to hurry off one leg and to spend most time on the other leg (often with accompanying asymmetry of arm movement). The type of antalgic gait may suggest the region that is involved. For example:

- Low back problem. Decreased rotation of the pelvis with the advancing leg results in a shortened step and caution when turning.
- Hip problem. The body 'bobs' over the painful side: fixed flexion may accentuate lumbar lordosis and exaggerate buttock prominence.
- Knee problem. Synovitis/deformity may prevent full extension during swing and soften heel strike. If the knee is held stiffly the body pivots around the leg during the stance phase and the leg is swung forward by circumduction.

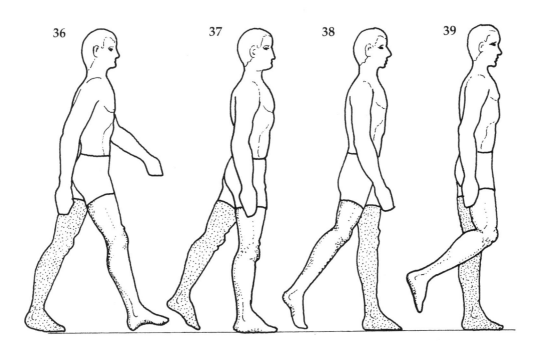

36–39 Principal phases of gait (nearest leg): (**36**) heel strike phase; (**37**) loading/stance phase; (**38**) toe-off; (**39**) swing phase.

- Hindfoot problem. With reduced ankle movement the leg may be externally rotated and slightly abducted. If the heel is painful, heel strike may be replaced by 'foot strike': the heel is kept off the floor and the knee does not fully extend. With Achilles tendon problems, push-off is avoided.
- Midfoot problem. The foot is held inverted (supinated) and push-off is from the lateral side.
- Forefoot problem. To prevent weight bearing on the forefoot the heel does not rise in late stance, and there is no push-off. The knee, hip, and trunk flex to maintain forward motion, and swing phase on the normal side is shortened, resulting in forward 'bobbing' during late stance on the painful side. Involvement of both forefeet combines to give a forward-leaning, short-stepped, shuffling gait.

Other abnormal (including neurological) gaits include:

- *Trendelenburg gait.* Due to ineffective hip abduction the pelvis drops down on the opposite side during stance phase on the affected side (**41**).
- *Waddling gait.* This is a bilateral Trendelenburg gait.
- *Hysterical/psychogenic gait.* Often variable, exaggerated or bizarre, conforming to no easily recognised pattern.
- *Spastic gait.* A narrow-based dragging gait; the patient has difficulty bending the knee, and the foot is raised by tilting the pelvis and swinging the leg forward in an arc of circumduction, with the toes scraping the ground.
- *High-stepping gait.* With a slap of the foot in the contact phase (due to unrestrained ankle plantar flexion) high-stepping gait occurs with weakness of tibialis anterior ('foot drop').
- *Wide-based stamping gait* (sensory ataxia). The patient suddenly raises the foot high and jerks it forward before bringing it to the ground with a stamp: the eyes are usually fixed to the ground to help compensate for loss of positional sense. Gait and balance are worsened by eye closure.
- *Wide-based staggering gait* (cerebellar ataxia). The feet are wide apart and placed irregularly; the arms are flung out to improve balance. Closing the eyes makes little difference.
- *Stooping, festinant gait* (parkinsonism). The arms do not swing; starting is slow, but after small shuffling steps the patient may break into a tottering run.

If the observed gait is entirely normal the patient is unlikely to have any major locomotor abnormality in the lower limbs or lumbar spine.

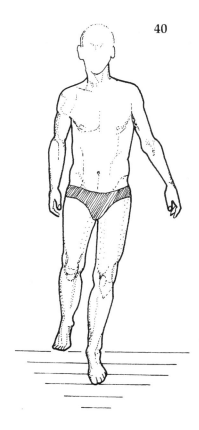

40 Antalgic gait.

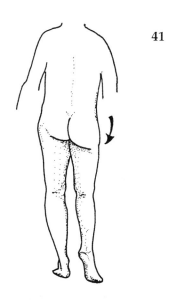

41 Trendelenburg gait.

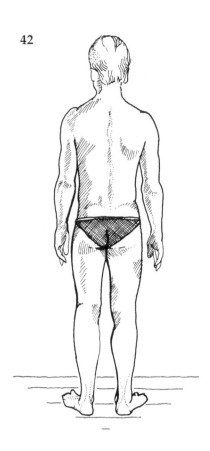

42

Inspection of the standing patient

Ask the patient to stand upright with arms outstretched by the sides.

Inspection from behind
Comparing one side with the other (**42**), look particularly for:

- A straight spine (no scoliosis/rib-cage asymmetry).
- Iliac crests at equal height.
- Normal muscle bulk/symmetry, especially of paraspinal, shoulder, and gluteal muscles.
- Popliteal swelling.
- Swelling/asymmetry around the Achilles tendons.
- Hindfoot deformity (valgus/varus).

While in this position apply point pressure to the midpoint of each supraspinatus (**43**), and undertake skin-fold rolling of the overlying skin (**44**), looking for increased tenderness suggestive of fibromyalgia.

42 Inspection of the standing patient from behind.

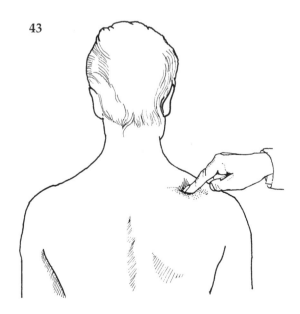

43

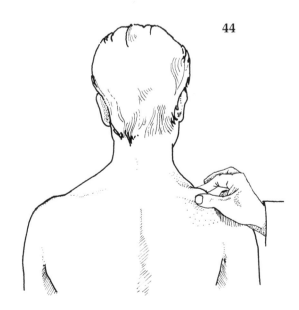

44

43 Applied pressure over midpoint of supraspinatus.

44 Skin-fold rolling (for fibromyalgia).

Inspection from the side

Look particularly for:

- Loss of normal cervical and lumbar lordosis, and alteration of normal mild thoracic kyphosis.
- Knee deformity (fixed flexion, genu recurvatum, posterior tibial subluxation).

While in this position (**45**), test lumbar spine and hip flexion by placing several fingers over the posterior spinous processes of the lower lumbar vertebrae and asking the patient to *'bend forwards and touch toes'* as best they can (**46**). The thoracolumbar spine should form a smooth curve and the palpating fingers move apart if the lumbar spine is normal: a good range of movement implies normal hip flexion.

Inspection from in front

Comparing one side with the other (**47**), look particularly for:

- Swelling, abnormal position, skin change over sternoclavicular and acromioclavicular joints.
- Equal shoulder height.
- Muscle wasting/asymmetry, especially of deltoids and quadriceps.
- Inability to fully extend elbows.
- Deformity (particularly varus, valgus) of knee.
- Deformity (particularly of hallux, MTPJs) of forefoot and alteration of foot arches (especially flat feet).

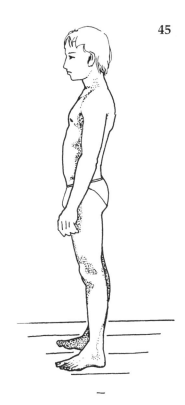

45   Inspection of the standing patient from the side.

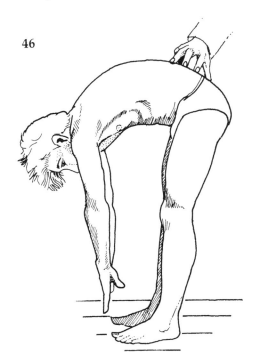

46   Inspection/palpation of patient attempting 'touching of toes'.

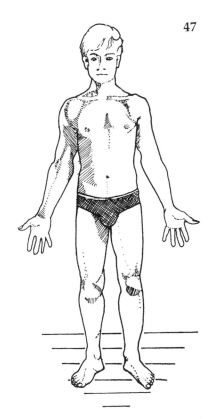

47   Inspection of the standing patient from in front.

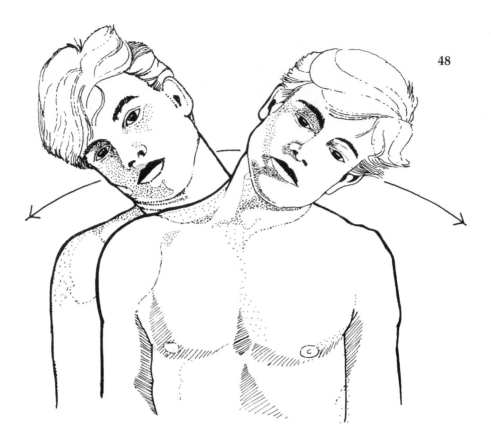

48 'Place your ear on your left, then right shoulder.'

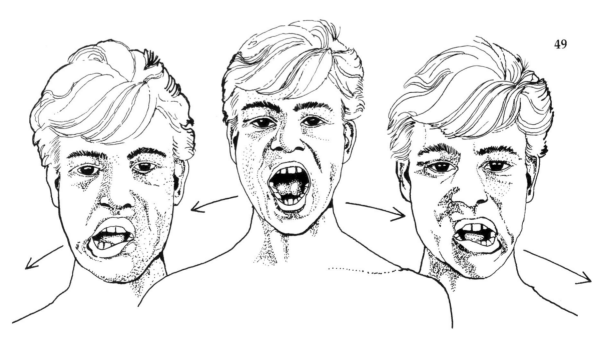

49 'Open your mouth wide, and move it from side to side.'

While in this position ask the patient to (1) *laterally flex the neck* to each side (**48**), and look for pain or restriction (lateral flexion is a sensitive test for cervical spine abnormality). (2) *Open the jaw wide and move it from side to side* (**49**). It should open easily, without deviation to either side. (3) *Place both hands behind the head* with the elbows back (**50**). External rotation and abduction are the earliest, most severely affected glenohumeral movements. Hands behind head also moves the acromioclavicular and sternoclavicular joints, and tests supraspinatus, infraspinatus, and teres minor. (4) *Place both hands out in front, palms down, fingers straight*, with elbows at 90° at the side (**51**). Inspect for abnormalities (particularly swelling, deformity, attitude, and skin changes) at distal radioulnar joint, wrists, MCPJs, and IPJs. Look for extensor tenosynovitis. (5) *Turn the hands over* (supination, **52**, testing proximal and distal radio-ulnar joints). Inspect the palmar aspects (particularly for wasting, skin changes, and flexor tenosynovitis swelling). (6) *Make a tight fist with*

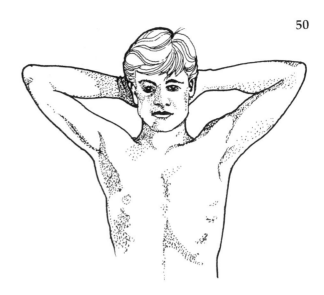

50 'Place your hands behind your head.'

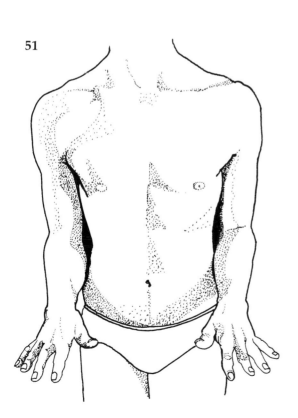

51 Inspect dorsal aspects of hands.

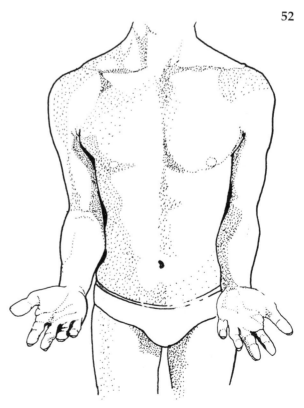

52 Inspect palmar aspects of hands.

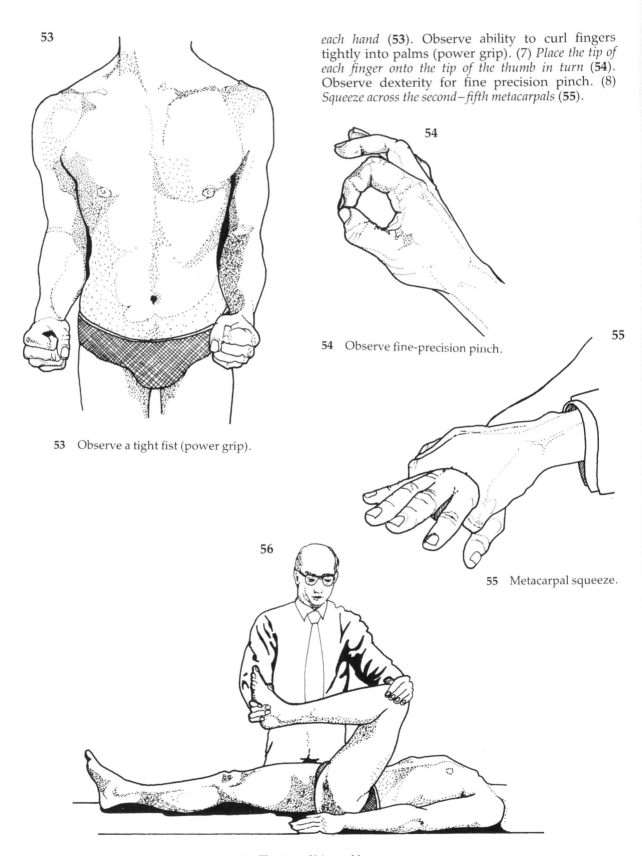

53

each hand (**53**). Observe ability to curl fingers tightly into palms (power grip). (7) *Place the tip of each finger onto the tip of the thumb in turn* (**54**). Observe dexterity for fine precision pinch. (8) *Squeeze across the second–fifth metacarpals* (**55**).

54

54 Observe fine-precision pinch.

53 Observe a tight fist (power grip).

55

55 Metacarpal squeeze.

56

56 Flexion of hip and knee.

Inspection/examination of the patient lying on a couch

Elderly patients, in particular, often find it uncomfortable to lie totally flat, and a sitting-up position is adequate for screening manoeuvres. With the patient reclining comfortably, the examiner should (1) *flex each hip and knee while holding the knee* (**56**). Ensure normal knee flexion and feel for crepitus. This again tests hip flexion. (2) *Passively internally rotate each hip* with the hip still flexed (**57**). This is a sensitive test for hip disease. (3) *Press on each patella and palpate for a balloon sign* (**58**). This tests the patellofemoral compartment and for synovitis in a joint commonly affected by all arthropathies. (4) *Squeeze all the metatarsals* (**59**) to test the MTPJs. (5) *Inspect the soles for callosities* (**60**).

If findings for all the above are normal it is very unlikely, with a negative locomotor history screen, that significant abnormalities are present.

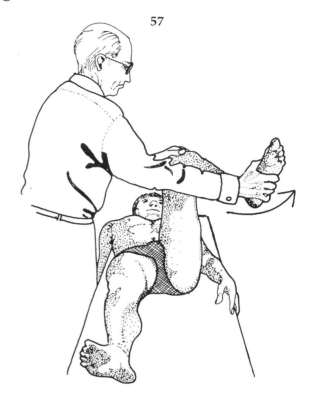

57

57 Internal rotation of the flexed hip.

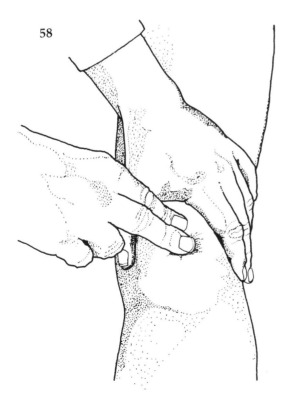

58

58 Patellofemoral stress test and palpation for balloon sign.

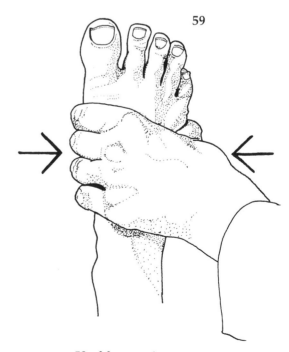

59

59 Metatarsal squeeze.

60

60 Inspection of soles.

RECORDING THE SCREEN

A useful shorthand for recording this screen in note form is the *'GALS'* template (*G* = gait, *A* = arms, *L* = legs, *S* = spine). If the appearance (**A**) and movement (**M**) of each component are normal, a tick is given:

		A		**M**
G	✔			
A		✔		✔
L		✔		✔
S		✔		✔

If abnormality is detected at one or more of these regions the tick is replaced by a cross, and further note of the abnormality is made. For example, in a patient with knee osteoarthritis:

		A		**M**
G	✗			
A		✔		✔
L		✗		✗
S		✔		✔

antalgic gait
R knee — varus
       ↓ flexion
    crepitus
    effusion

SUMMARY OF SCREENING EXAMINATION

(1) Inspection of the patient walking, turning, and walking back
(2) Inspection of the patient standing
    (a) from behind
        press over mid-supraspinatus
        skin-fold rolling
    (b) from the side
        'touch toes' (lumbar flexion)
    (c) from the front
        'ear on shoulder' (lateral cervical flexion)
        'open jaw, move side to side' (TMJs)
        'hands behind head' (glenohumeral)
        inspect dorsum of hands
        observe supination of hands, inspect palms
        'make a fist' (power grip)
        'touch fingers on thumb' (precision pinch)
        metacarpal squeeze
(3) Examination of the patient lying on a couch
    feel knee crepitus during knee/hip flexion
    internal rotation of hip in flexion
    balloon sign at knee
    metatarsal squeeze
    inspect soles

3 Hand

FUNCTION

The wrist and hand, each comprising many small joints, act as a single functional unit. The hand undertakes a variety of important functions including:

1 *Grip and manipulation.* The two important basic grips are:

- *Fine precision pinch* (**61**). This is achieved by opposing the pulp surfaces of the thumb and finger (usually the index finger), and requires rotation of the thumb (and to some extent finger) during opposition. 'Scissors' pinch is less precise opposition of the thumb against the side of the index finger.
- *Power grip* (**62**). Achieved by curling the fingers tight into the palm, the power grip is optimised by extension and locking of the wrist (permitting full power from the finger flexors). The grip is maximal with 90° rotation and 45° ulnar deviation ('hammering' position). The hook grip is a modification of the power configuration.

A range of variants can be generated from these basic grips, giving the hand great flexibility for manipulation. Grip is enhanced by complementary use of both hands, and impaired function in one hand may reduce overall function considerably.

2 *Proprioception.* Hands are the principal point of contact for touch sensitivity with the environment.

3 *Communication.* Hands undertake a range of non-verbal signals and are important in social contact (e.g. hand shakes, caresses).

4 *Locomotion,* e.g. during crawling, swimming.

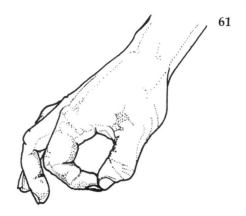

61 Fine precision pinch.

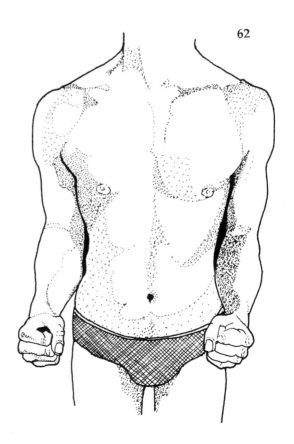

62 Power grip.

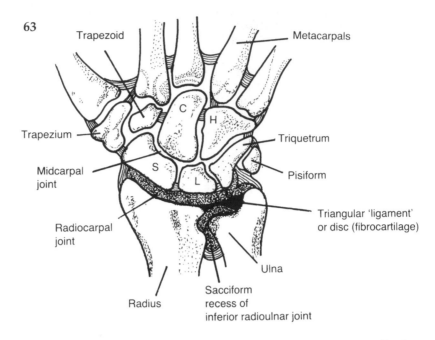

63 Bones and joints of the wrist (S = scaphoid, L = lunate, C = capitate, H = hamate).

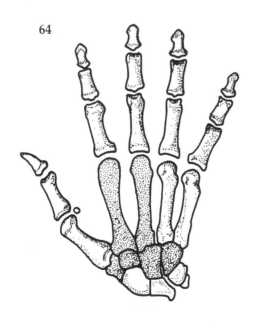

64 The L-shaped immobile segment.

The *inferior radioulnar joint* (**63**) is delineated distally by the triangular disc or 'ligament' (a key stabiliser to the wrist). The capsule and synovium extend proximally between the radius and the ulnar as the sacciform recess. Together with the superior radioulnar joint it permits supination/flexion.

The *radiocarpal joint*, with its separate synovial cavity, permits flexion, extension and lateral movement between the radius (and triangular ligament) and the proximal row of the carpus (scaphoid, lunate, triquetrum). The *midcarpal joint* has a separate synovial space (often communicating with carpometacarpal cavities) and connects the proximal and distal rows (trapezium, trapezoid, capitate, hamate): only minor movement (flexion, extension, some rotation) occurs here. The second and third *carpometacarpal joints* (CMCJs) permit little if any movement; the second and third metacarpals and distal carpal row thus form a fixed L-shaped unit (**64**) around which, in functional terms, the rest of the hand is built. The first CMCJ is exceptionally mobile: the metacarpal sits astride the trapezium, facing the ulnar border. The fourth and fifth CMCJs are less mobile than the first but move together on the hamate, permitting formation of a 'hollow palm'.

The *metacarpophalangeal joints* (MCPJs: **65**) are modified hinge joints: their position is marked on the palmar surface by the distal palmar crease. Each proximal phalanx base has a cartilaginous volar extension (the palmar ligament or plate). The deep transverse metacarpal ligament joins the second to fifth volar plates (**66**). Each MCPJ has a radial and ulnar lateral ligament eccentrically placed across the joint, tightening only in flexion (**67**).

The *proximal* and *distal interphalangeal joints* (PIPJs, DIPJs) are true hinge joints. They also possess palmar plates, and fibrous tunnels occur on the palmar aspects of the phalanges. Each inter-phalangeal joint (IPJ) has radial and ulnar collateral ligaments centrally placed across the joint (tight in both flexion and extension). The synovium of each MCPJ and IPJ extends more proximally than distally (**65**) due to the arrangement of tendon slips and other structures which cause progressive tightening of space distally.

The hand is primarily designed for flexion (gripping). The long flexor tendons (**68**) run in the common flexor tendon sheath (flexor pollicis longus often has a separate sheath): all are encased by the flexor retinaculum. The palmar fascia (an extension of palmaris longus) attaches to the flexor retinaculum and partly divides into four, attaching to the deep transverse metacarpal ligament and phalanges. The median nerve passes tight alongside the flexor tendons beneath the retinaculum in the *carpal tunnel* (it may thus be compressed by tenosynovitis). The extensor tendons are also long structures enclosed by the

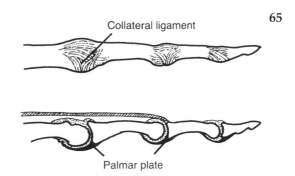

65

Collateral ligament

Palmar plate

65 Metacarpophalangeal and interphalangeal joints.

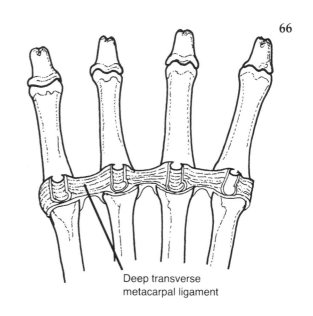

66

Deep transverse metacarpal ligament

66 Volar plate arrangement.

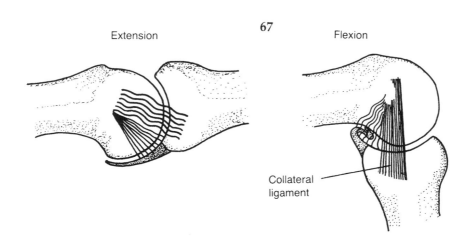

67

Extension

Flexion

Collateral ligament

67 Tightening of MCPJ collateral ligaments in flexion.

extensor retinaculum (**69**). Extensor pollicis brevis and abductor pollicis longus are encased in a separate fibrous canal at the radial styloid region where inflammation may give rise to stenosing tenovaginitis (*de Quervain's tenosynovitis*).

Wrist and hand joints are commonly involved in inflammatory conditions (e.g. rheumatoid, sero-negative spondarthropathy). Generalised osteo-arthritis predominantly involves DIPJs and PIPJs, the first CMCJ and the scapho-trapezoid joint (other carpal joints are spared). Isolated involvement of radiocarpal and midcarpal joints is common in crystal-associated arthropathy (pyro-phosphate arthropathy and gout).

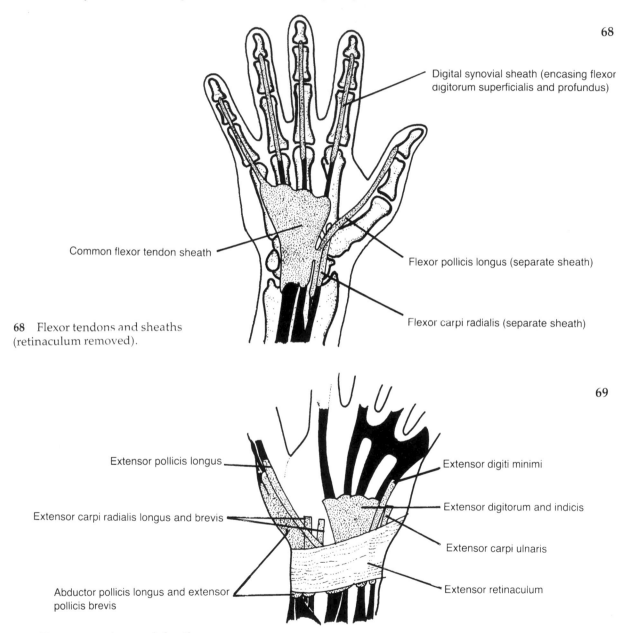

68

Digital synovial sheath (encasing flexor digitorum superficialis and profundus)

Common flexor tendon sheath

Flexor pollicis longus (separate sheath)

Flexor carpi radialis (separate sheath)

68   Flexor tendons and sheaths (retinaculum removed).

69

Extensor pollicis longus

Extensor carpi radialis longus and brevis

Abductor pollicis longus and extensor pollicis brevis

Extensor digiti minimi

Extensor digitorum and indicis

Extensor carpi ulnaris

Extensor retinaculum

69   Extensor tendons and sheaths.

SYMPTOMS

Pain from any of the small joints in the wrist and hand is usually well localised and the patient easily pinpoints its source. However, three common conditions may cause radiation of pain on the radial side of the hand (**70–72**):

- *First CMCJ arthropathy* (usually osteoarthritis). This is the one joint that may cause wide

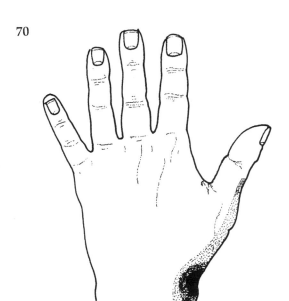

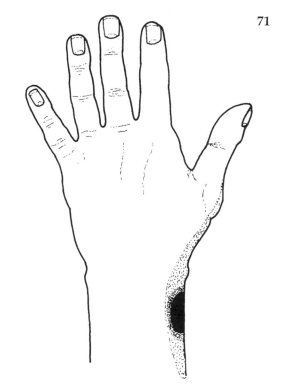

70–72 Pain radiation in (**70**) first carpometacarpal joint arthropathy, (**71**) de Quervain's tenosynovitis, and (**72**) carpal tunnel syndrome.

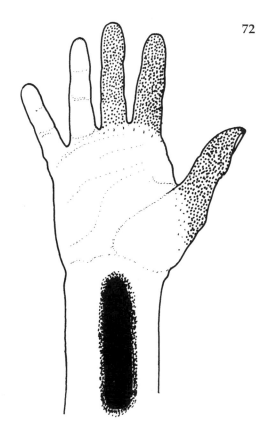

72

radiation (distally up the thumb, proximally up the distal forearm), though pain is maximal over the joint itself.

- *De Quervain's tenosynovitis.* Pain is maximal around the radial styloid but often radiates into the thumb and proximally up the forearm.
- *Carpal tunnel syndrome.* The key symptom suggesting peripheral nerve entrapment is *nocturnal or early morning exacerbation of symptoms* (symptoms may be confined to this time). In carpal tunnel syndrome, median nerve compression may cause (1) paraesthesia and dysaesthesia distally to the thumb, index and middle fingers, often with clumsiness, and (2) painful aching proximally up the forearm, occasionally to the elbow.

Problems (particularly synovitis) affecting hand joints are often very apparent to the patient, due to early interference with activities of daily living (dressing, etc.): even mild tenosynovitis or IPJ synovitis may cause tightness of rings.

Pain and sensory disturbance may radiate into the hand from above, particularly the elbow (arthritis, epicondylitis), shoulder (arthropathy, rotator cuff), and cervical spine (root entrapment of C6, 7, 8). In these situations symptoms are often less well defined and accompanied by more proximal symptoms.

INSPECTION AT REST

Inspect and compare the dorsal and palmar surfaces of both hands, then inspect from the side with hands outstretched.

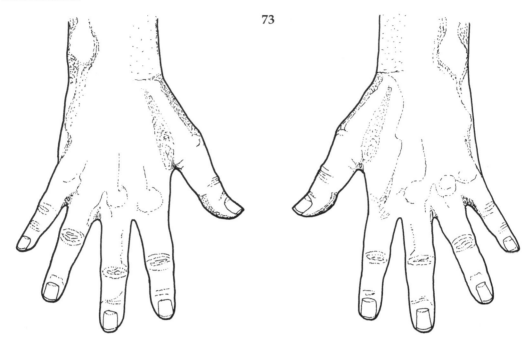

73

73 Inspection of the back of the hands.

Inspection of the extensor surface

Inspect the back of the hands rested on the patient's lap or on a flat surface (**73**). Look for:

Skin and nail changes

These include erythema, psoriasis, vitiligo, mixed hyper/hypopigmentation ('salt and pepper' appearance of scleroderma), skin tightness with loss of flexures (*sclerodactyly*: typical of scleroderma and overlap connective tissue syndromes); and current or past evidence of trauma. Violaceous/silvery raised lesions (*Gottron's papules*) occur over extensor surfaces in dermatomyositis. Lupus rashes often affect skin *between* joints, vasculitic rashes often affect lateral more than dorsal aspects of fingers. The nails require inspection for clubbing, thimble pitting, splinter haemorrhages, subungual hyperkeratosis, dystrophy and abnormalities of nailfold capillaries.

Swelling

All joint swellings are most prominent on the dorsal surface. Radiocarpal synovitis (**74**) produces

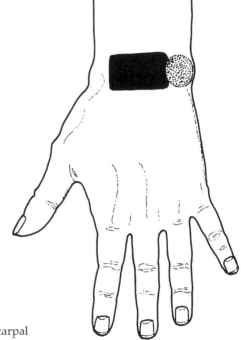

74

74 Position and shape of swelling due to radiocarpal (black) and inferior radioulnar (stippled) synovitis.

rectangular swelling symmetrically placed each side of the joint line; inferior radioulnar synovitis causes a domed swelling that rounds off the distal ulna prominence; intercarpal and CMCJ synovitis usually produce modest swelling centred over their joint lines. However, both MCPJ and IPJ synovitis cause swelling more proximal than distal to the joint line (75), MCPJ synovitis producing swelling between the metacarpal heads, and IPJ swelling producing posterolateral bulging between the extensor tendon above and the lateral collateral ligaments on each side. With moderate–gross IPJ swelling, stretching of the skin makes the overlying wrinkles less distinct. Extensor tenosynovitis also produces swelling over the carpus: it may differ from radiocarpal synovitis in being asymmetrically spread across the joint line, extending more distally over the metacarpals and having an irregular distal contour (76).

Deformity

A variety of deformities may occur, all best seen from the dorsal aspect. Apart from synovitis, undue prominence of the ulnar styloid may result from subluxation caused by weakening and rupture of the distal radioulnar ligament (usually rheumatoid). Conversely, the ulnar prominence may not be apparent, due to erosive disease or previous surgery. Osteophytosis of the first CMCJ may cause 'squaring' of the hand (77). *Ulnar deviation* at MCPJs (78) usually accompanies and follows radial deviation at the wrist (usually rheumatoid). *Volar subluxation* of phalanges at MCPJs leads to prominence of metacarpal heads and a step-down deformity. Lateral deviation (radial or ulnar) at IPJs (77), and firm posterolateral swellings of DIPJs (*Heberden's nodes*) and PIPJs (*Bouchard's nodes*) are characteristic of osteoarthritis. Combined deformities include 'swan neck' (PIPJ hyperextension, DIPJ hyperflexion: 79), 'boutonniere' ('buttonhole': PIPJ hyperflexion, DIPJ hyperextension — the PIPJ pushing through the extensor tendon like a button through a buttonhole — 80), and 'Z' deformity of the thumb (MCPJ hyperflexion, IPJ hyperextension: 81). Inability to place the fingers flat (fixed flexion) can result from flexor tendon or joint problems.

Wasting

This is often difficult to observe. Apart from wasting of dorsal interosseus muscles, marked 'guttering' between extensor tendons may result from volar subluxation of the carpus, which automatically makes the extensor tendons and gaps between them more prominent.

Attitude

The way the patient holds the hand may suggest the degree of pain and discomfort. With synovitis of any hand/wrist joints the patient is most comfortable in mild flexion.

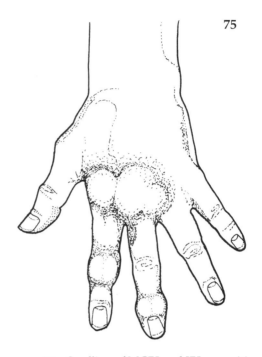

75 Swelling of MCPJ and IPJ synovitis.

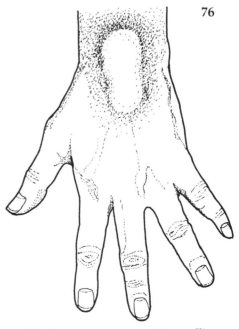

76 Extensor tenosynovitis swelling.

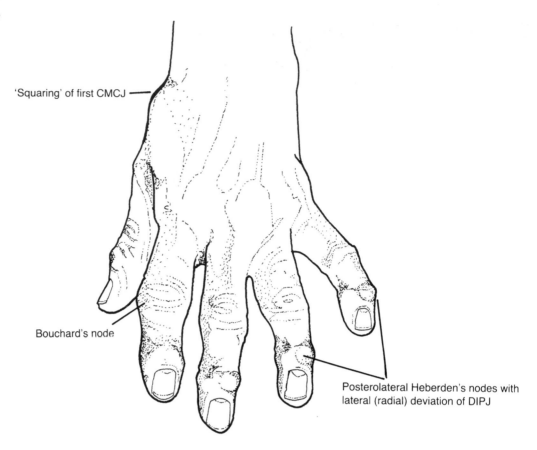

'Squaring' of first CMCJ

Bouchard's node

Posterolateral Heberden's nodes with lateral (radial) deviation of DIPJ

77 Typical hand deformities in generalised osteoarthritis.

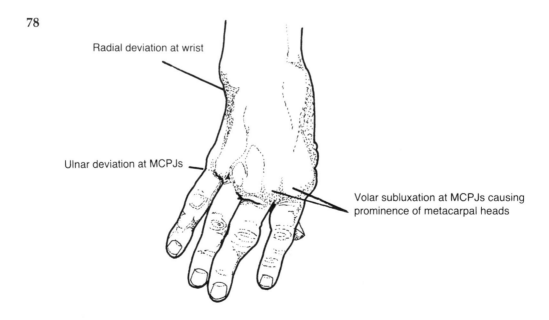

Radial deviation at wrist

Ulnar deviation at MCPJs

Volar subluxation at MCPJs causing prominence of metacarpal heads

78 Ulnar deviation at MCPJs accompanying radial deviation at the wrist.

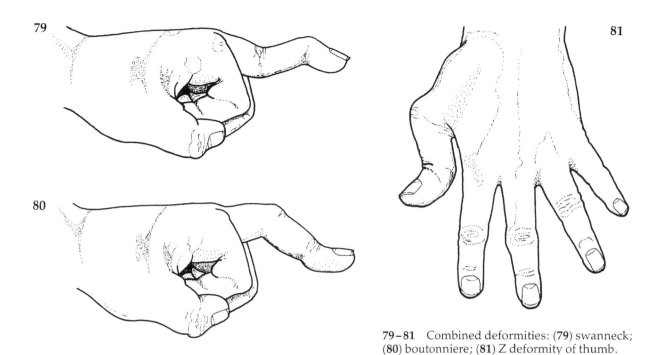

79–81 Combined deformities: (79) swanneck; (80) boutonniere; (81) Z deformity of thumb.

Inspection of the palmar surface

Ask the patient to pronate the hands. Difficulty or pain during pronation reflects problems with the superior and/or inferior radioulnar joints. Supination/pronation involves the radius moving over the stationary ulna: if the radioulnar joints are compromised the patient may use a trick manoeuvre (82, 83), bringing the elbow across the abdomen to increase supination (by partly rotating the ulna).

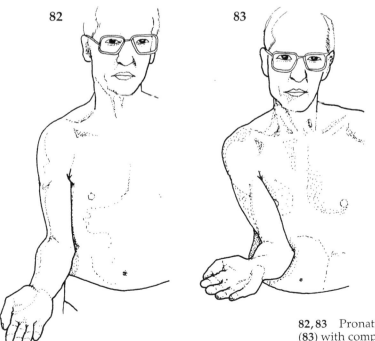

82,83 Pronation with flexed elbow: (82) normal; (83) with compromised radioulnar joints.

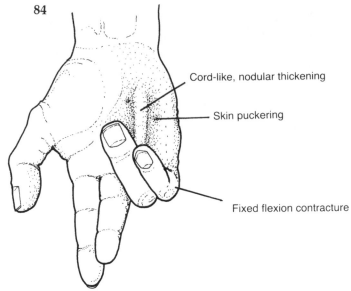

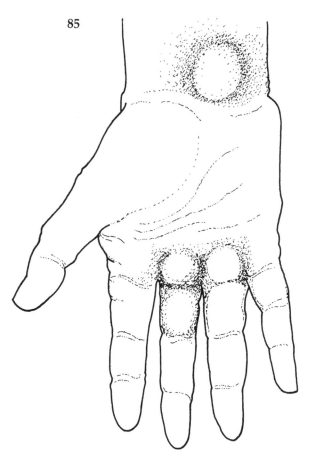

84   Cord-like, nodular thickening

    Skin puckering

    Fixed flexion contracture

84   Dupuytren's contracture.

On the palmar surface look for:

Skin changes
Palmar erythema is common in rheumatoid disease. *Dupuytren's contracture* is recognised as puckering of the skin with thickening of the palmar fascia: in established cases there may be fixed flexion contracture, predominantly affecting the ring and little fingers (**84**). *Small vessel infarcts* often occur as black spots, particularly on finger pulps.

Swelling
Swelling on the volar aspect most commonly represents flexor tenosynovitis, often most obvious proximal to the wrist crease, between the distal palmar crease and finger base, and occasionally between the skin creases of the fingers (**85**). As a result of the thick flexor apparatus, joint swelling is rarely apparent on the palmar surface.

Wasting
Unlike the dorsal surface the palms are an excellent site to observe muscle wasting. Irrespective of age, both thenar and hypothenar eminences should be convex. Localised outer thenar wasting usually reflects median nerve compression: it often also accompanies first CMCJ arthritis.

85   Flexor tenosynovitis swelling.

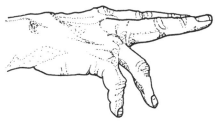

86 Complete extensor tendon rupture (ring finger and little finger).

Lateral inspection

Ask the patient to outstretch the hands and inspect from the side. The main features to note are:

Ability to fully extend fingers

The patient may have almost no active extension of one or more fingers (commonly the little finger and the ring finger: **86**). The examiner, however, may be able to extend the finger passively, only to see it drop down when the finger is released. This combination reflects *extensor tendon rupture* (in inflammatory disease this usually occurs close to the ulnar styloid). Some patients have *partial* active, but full passive, extension: this reflects rupture of the extensor tendon slips, permitting the extensor tendon to drop to the ulnar side of the MCPJ. Sometimes the *slipped extensor tendon* can be palpated and pushed onto its usual position above the MCPJ: if the examiner holds it there, the patient may be able to fully extend the finger only for it to return to the original situation when the examiner lets go (**87, 88**).

Volar subluxation of the carpus

This produces a 'dinner fork' deformity (**89**: perhaps the most characteristic hand deformity of rheumatoid).

Swelling over dorsum of wrist

This may have been noted earlier, reflecting synovitis (radiocarpal, midcarpal) or extensor tenosynovitis. To differentiate tendon sheath from joint swelling, inspect the swelling with the MCPJs flexed; then ask the patient to fully extend the fingers (**90**). Tenosynovial swelling moves proximally with the tendons, its distal boundary becoming more definite as the tenosynovium 'tucks' in (the 'tuck' or 'shelf' sign). Joint swelling remains unaltered by extensor tendon movement.

Volar subluxation at the MCPJs

This may be more obvious from the lateral view (see **78**).

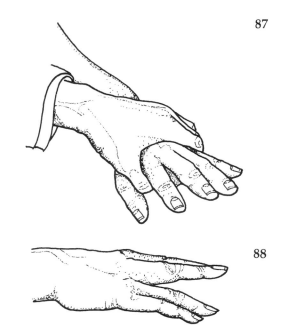

87,88 Extensor tendon slip. In (**87**) the examiner can correct the slip, permitting full finger extension. When the examiner lets go (**88**) the fingers drop again.

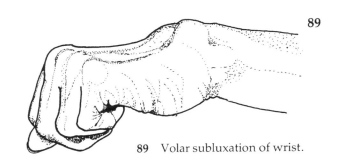

89 Volar subluxation of wrist.

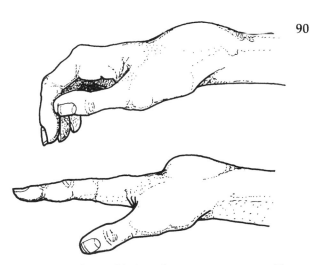

90 The 'tuck' sign of extensor tenosynovitis.

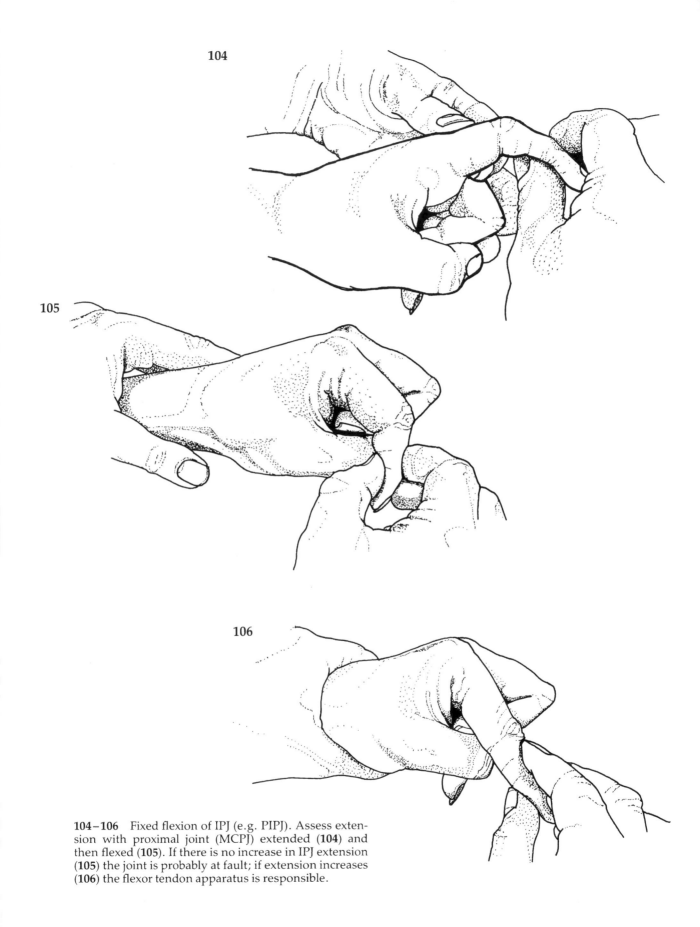

104

105

106

104–106 Fixed flexion of IPJ (e.g. PIPJ). Assess extension with proximal joint (MCPJ) extended (**104**) and then flexed (**105**). If there is no increase in IPJ extension (**105**) the joint is probably at fault; if extension increases (**106**) the flexor tendon apparatus is responsible.

ADDITIONAL TESTS

Stability of small joints

Stability of IPJs is tested by holding the phalanx each side of the joint and moving one laterally while the other is held in position. Normally there is little lateral movement, irrespective of whether the IPJ is flexed or extended. Stability of MCPJs is tested by forced lateral movement while the MCPJ is fully flexed (MCPJ collateral ligaments tighten only in flexion — in extension, they are lax and permit marked lateral movement).

Fixed flexion of IPJ

To determine whether this results from problems with the flexor tendon apparatus or with the capsule/joint itself, assess the degree of flexion with the proximal joint in full extension (**104**). Then flex the proximal joint, relaxing the flexor tendons (**105**), and again assess the range of movement in the joint of interest. If there is now more movement than before (**106**) it suggests that the flexor tendon apparatus is primarily at fault. If, however, the range of movement is equally reduced with the proximal joint flexed or extended, it is more likely that restriction is due to capsular/joint damage.

De Quervain's tenosynovitis

In this condition a localised area of tenderness may be detected in a line along the lateral border of the distal radius. This may be accompanied by increased temperature and linear soft-tissue swelling. A useful stress test is to ask the patient to grasp the thumb in the palm while the examiner cautiously performs passively lateral flexion to the ulnar side (**107**). This manoeuvre can be uncomfortable in normal individuals but in de Quervain's tenosynovitis it causes marked pain (Finkelstein's test).

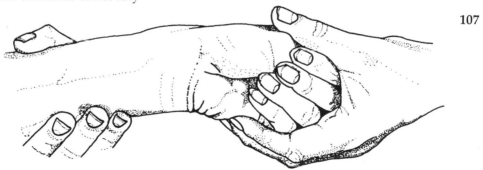

107

107 Finkelstein's test.

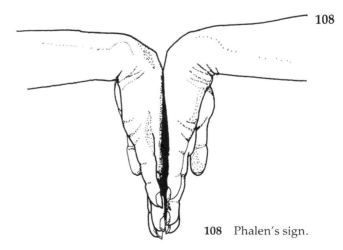

108

Carpal tunnel syndrome

The median nerve gives off a sensory branch (supplying skin on the radial side of the palm) above the wrist before it passes through the carpal tunnel. Compression in the tunnel therefore causes numbness/dysaesthesia and altered sensation only in the thumb, index and middle fingers. The patient's symptoms may be reproduced (1) by percussion over the anterior wrist distal to the proximal skin crease (*Tinel's sign*), or (2) by asking the patient to sustain forced flexion of the wrist for at least 1 min (*Phalen's test*; **108**).

108 Phalen's sign.

The median supplies the lateral two lumbricals, opponens pollicis, abductor pollicis brevis and flexor pollicis brevis ('LOAF'). To determine early weakness, test abductor pollicis brevis (always median nerve supply) by asking the patient to raise the thumb vertically from a flat supinated hand against resistance, feeling the muscle as it contracts (**109**). Later diminution of thumb opposition power is tested by asking the patient to oppose the thumb and index finger as the examiner tries to pull through the loop with an index finger. Wasting of abductor brevis and opponens may cause conspicuous hollowing of the outer thenar eminence.

Ulnar nerve lesion

Compression is usually at the elbow but may also occur (± combined carpal tunnel syndrome) at the wrist as the nerve passes through Guyon's canal (formed by the pisohamate ligament bridging the pisiform and hamate). The ulnar gives off two sensory branches above the wrist (supplying the palmar and dorsal surfaces of the hand): therefore, compression in Guyon's canal causes altered sensation only in the little and ring fingers (± small muscle changes).

For early ulnar nerve lesions look for weakness (± wasting) of the first dorsal interosseous: with the hand flat, ask the patient to abduct the index finger against resistance, comparing one side with the other. Later weakness of all dorsal interossei and abductor digiti minimi (ulnar nerve; C8, T1) and all palmar interossei (ulnar nerve; C8, T1) leads to weak abduction and adduction of the second–fifth fingers. To test these movements the hand must be flat since the long extensors and flexors act to some extent as abductors and adductors (**110**). Apart from resisted active movements, adduction can be tested by trying to remove a strip of paper held between the patient's adducted fingers. Adductor pollicis brevis is also supplied by the ulnar nerve and may be tested by asking the patient to grasp a piece of paper between the adducted thumb and index finger: as the examiner attempts to pull the paper away the terminal phalanx of the thumb will flex due to weakness of the adductor and unopposed pull of the flexor pollicis longus (Froment's sign: **111**, **112**).

Radial nerve lesion

This causes weak wrist dorsiflexion if mild, wrist drop if severe, with wasting of the forearm muscles. Sensory loss on the dorsum of the hand is minimal.

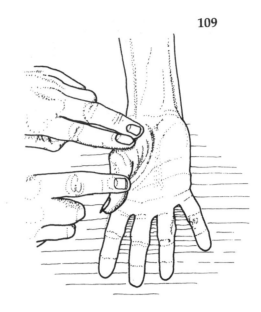

109 Testing abductor pollicis brevis.

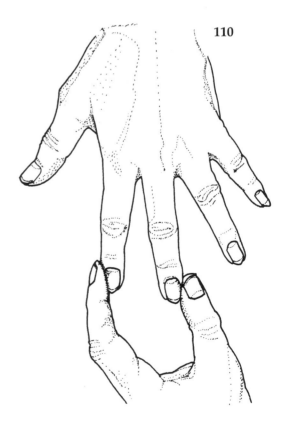

110 Testing finger abduction.

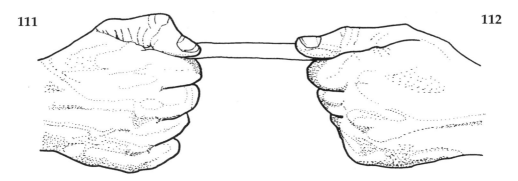

111,112 Froment's sign: **(111)** positive (thumb flexes); **(112)** normal (thumb adducts).

SUMMARY OF EXAMINATION OF THE HAND

(1) Inspection at rest
    (a) dorsal surface
        skin, nail changes
        swelling (joint synovitis, tenosynovitis)
        deformity
        wasting
        attitude
    (b) palmar surface
        skin changes (erythema, Dupuytren's)
        swelling (tenosynovitis)
        wasting
    (c) from side, fingers outstretched
        tendon rupture, slip
        deformity (volar subluxation of the wrist and MCPJs)
        wrist swelling (tuck sign)
(2) Inspection during usage
    (a) power grip
    (b) fine precision pinch
(3) Palpation
    (a) increased warmth
    (b) each joint in turn (swelling, joint-line tenderness, crepitus, movement)
        radiocarpal joint
        inferior radioulnar joint
        second–fifth MCPJs (+ metacarpal squeeze, flexor tendon sheath crepitus)
        second–fifth IPJs (+ flexor tendon sheath crepitus)
        thumb joints: first CMCJ, MCPJ, IPJ

4 Elbow

The primary role of the elbow is to permit accurate spatial positioning of the hand. The elbow anchors the strong flexors and extensors of the wrist and hand, and once the shoulder has grossly directed the arm, elbow movements permit fine adjustment to limb height and length. In addition, forearm rotation (at elbow and wrist) helps place the hand in the most effective functional position.

Heavy demands on forearm muscles and poor soft-tissue protection make the elbow particularly prone to enthesopathy and bursitis. Although not uncommonly involved in inflammatory arthropathies (e.g. rheumatoid), the elbow is an uncommon target site for arthritis other than haemophilia and syringomyelia-associated Charcot arthropathy. Primary osteoarthritis is distinctly unusual.

FUNCTIONAL ANATOMY

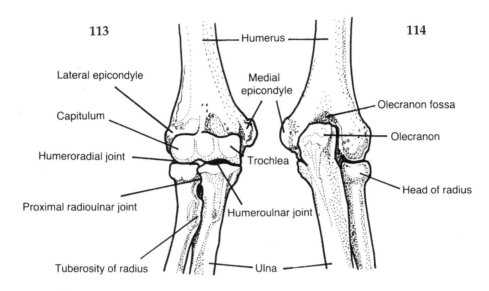

113, 114 The elbow joint: (**113**) anterior view; (**114**) posterior view.

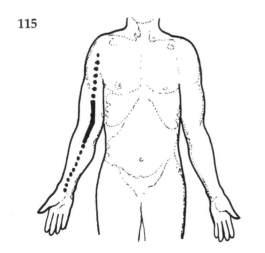

115 Extension of the elbow, showing 'carrying angle'.

The elbow is a compound joint comprising three articulations: the humeroulnar and humeroradial joints (permitting flexion/extension) and the proximal radioulnar joint (which, with the humeroradial and inferior radioulnar joints, permits rotation: **113, 114**).

The *humeroulnar ('trochlea') joint* forms a uniaxial hinge between the trochlea of the humerus and the ulna trochlea notch. When the elbow is fully flexed (about 145°) the longitudinal axes of the upper arm and forearm are parallel; however, due to the shape of the trochlea, as the arm extends in the anatomical position (palms forward) the upper arm and forearm form a valgus 'carrying angle' at the elbow (**115**). This is wider in females (10–15°) than in males (5°) and may be increased (cubitus valgus) as a developmental abnormality (e.g. part of Turner's syndrome).

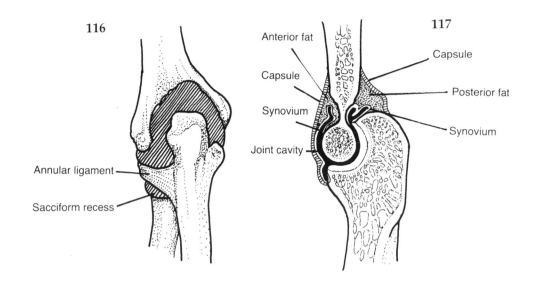

116, 117 Synovial outline of the elbow: (**116**) posterior view; (**117**) section through the joint.

The *humeroradial joint* is a modified uniaxial hinge (allowing rotation and flexion/extension), corresponding to a ball and socket between the capitulum of the humerus and the concave fovea of the radial head: during supination/pronation the radial head revolves on the capitulum. The *superior radioulnar joint* comprises the pivot between the proximal rim of the radial head and the ulnar radial notch, together with the cartilage-lined annular ligament that encircles the radial head. The strong interosseous membrane of the fore-arm prevents parallel displacement of the ulna and the radius and transmits longitudinal stresses from one bone to the other.

The three joints share a common capsule (**116, 117**). On the radius the capsule extends as the sacciform recess beneath the annular ligament. Large intracapsular fat pads lie in the three fossae of the humerus, buttressing against extremes of movement. Stability is afforded by the shape of the trochlear joint, the annular ligament, and the cord-like radial and fan-shaped ulnar collateral ligaments (**118, 119**). The latter, together with flexor carpi ulnaris, form the cubital tunnel through which the ulnar nerve passes.

The axis of flexion/extension runs through the two epicondyles: muscles in front of this axis act as flexors, those behind as extensors. Many of the muscles act on several joints — their action at the

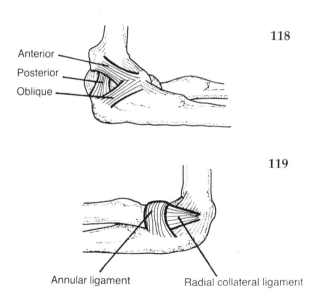

118, 119 Ligaments around the elbow: (**118**) the three portions of the fan-shaped medial ligament; (**119**) the lateral ligament.

elbow varies according to the attitude of neighbouring joints. Principal elbow flexors (**120–122**) are the biceps (inserting into the radial tuberosity, thus supinating as well as flexing: **120**), the brachialis (a short pure flexor: **121**), and the brachioradialis (a flexor with the forearm in neutral rotation: **122**). The principal elbow extensor is the triceps, joining the scapula (long head) and humerus (medial, lateral heads) to the olecranon (**123**). Pronation is principally via the pronator teres (the anterior interosseous nerve passes between its two heads) and the pronator quadratus. Although the biceps is the strongest supinator in flexion, the supinator muscle acts in any flexion/extension position (in 30% of people the posterior interosseous nerve passes through the fibrous arcade of Frohse between the two heads of the supinator and may rarely become compressed — *'radial tunnel syndrome'* — causing weakness of the forearm extensors but no sensory loss).

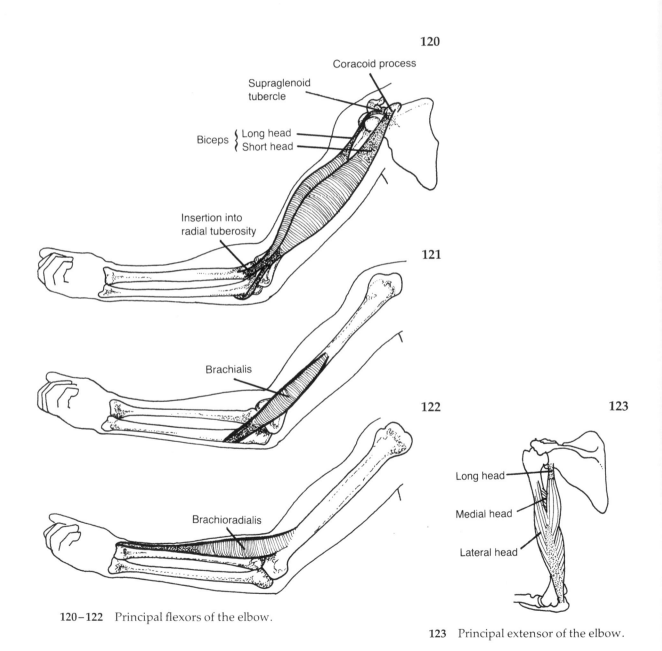

120–122 Principal flexors of the elbow.

123 Principal extensor of the elbow.

Normal active flexion is about 145° from the fully extended position: passive flexion often achieves another 10–15°. The elbow hyperextends 10° in many normal women (more in the hypermobility syndrome). Muscular individuals may lack 10° at each end of the range.

The bones and ligaments around the elbow anchor the forearm muscles. The origins of extensores carpi radialis brevis and longus ('fist clenchers') at the lateral epicondyle (with the brachioradialis origin just above) are the usual site of pain in 'lateral epicondylitis' (**124, 125**). Both muscles are weak elbow flexors but principally extend the wrist, optimising the action of the flexors in the power grip. The common tendon insertion at the medial epicondyle (for pronator teres, flexor carpi radialis, palmaris longus, and flexor carpi ulnaris) is, similarly, the site of pain in 'medial epicondylitis' (**126**).

Several bursae, none communicating with the joint, occur around the elbow, the largest being the superficial olecranon bursa overlying the olecranon prominence.

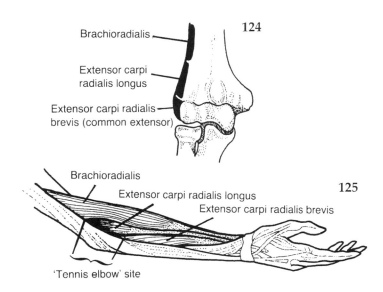

124, 125 Tendon insertions around the lateral epicondyle.

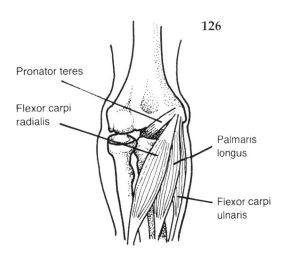

126 Tendon insertions around the medial epicondyle.

SYMPTOMS

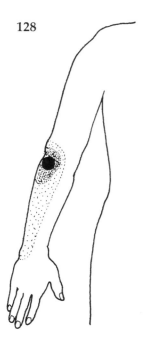

127 Site of pain radiation from the elbow joint.

Pain from the three elbow compartments is usually felt maximally at the elbow, close to its origin: severe arthropathy may cause radiation of pain down the forearm and, to a lesser extent, proximally to the upper arm (**127**). Pain of lateral epicondylitis ('tennis elbow') is usually maximal close to the epicondyle, radiating down the outer aspect of the forearm towards the wrist (**128**): it is particularly marked during power grip with the wrist extended. Medial epicondylitis ('golfer's elbow') causes pain maximum around the medial epicondyle, radiating down the flexor aspect of the forearm towards the wrist (**129**). Pain from olecranon bursitis is well localised, usually showing no clear relationship to passive or resisted elbow movement: it may be provoked by leaning the elbow on a table, or on flexion at the elbow when tight clothing is worn.

Four dermatomes cover sensation around the elbow (**130**). Pain referred from above is usually ill-defined at the elbow, with the site of maximum intensity elsewhere: it may originate from glenohumeral or rotator cuff lesions or from root entrapment (C5 or C6; less commonly, T1 or T2). Pain may refer up towards the elbow from de Quervain's tenosynovitis, carpal tunnel syndrome or, rarely, severe wrist arthropathy.

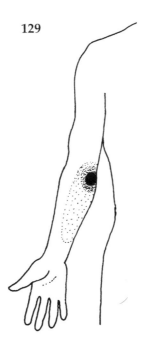

128 Pain pattern in lateral epicondylitis.

129 Pain pattern in medial epicondylitis.

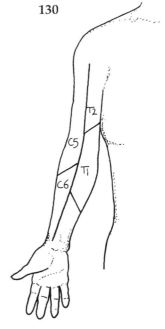

130 Dermatomes around the elbow.

EXAMINATION

Inspect from in front and from behind with the patient's arm hanging by the side; then inspect during active flexion, extension, and supination/pronation; then palpate.

Inspection at rest

From behind (131) the most prominent feature is the olecranon process: para-olecranon grooves separate this from the epicondyles, the medial epicondyle being more prominent than the lateral (the three bony prominences form a straight line with the elbow extended). *From in front* the triangular cubital fossa (132) forms a hollow bounded superiorly by the biceps and its tendon, medially by the pronator teres and the common flexors, laterally by the brachioradialis, and the floor comprising the brachialis muscle and tendon (+ joint capsule and supinator). The fossa contains the brachial artery and veins, the median and musculo-cutaneous nerves, and, superficially, the median cubital vein (joining the medially placed basilic to the cephalic vein).

With the patient's arms extended by the side, examine from in front and then from behind for the following.

Skin changes
For example, erythema (confined in bursitis or over the whole joint) and scars: the extensor aspect is a common site for psoriasis, nodules, and pressure sores (133).

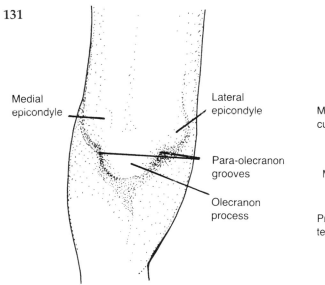

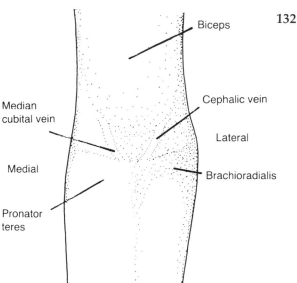

131 Surface landmarks of the elbow — posterior view.

132 Surface landmarks of the elbow — anterior view.

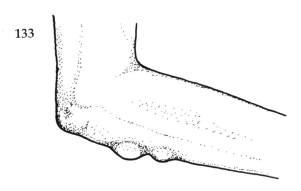

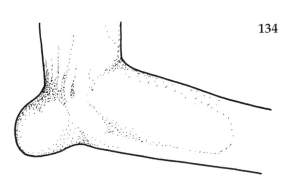

133 Nodules around the elbow.

134 Olecranon bursitis.

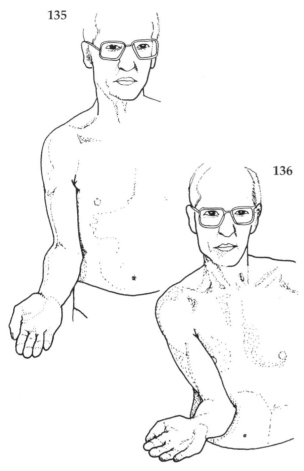

135

136

135, 136 Supination with flexed elbow: (**135**) normal; (**136**) trick manoeuvre (limited supination).

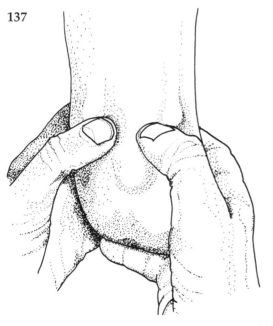

137

137 Palpation of the elbow (posterior approach).

Swelling
Synovial swelling is most apparent over the radial head anteriorly, and over the para-olecranon grooves posteriorly (medial > lateral): if marked, the whole elbow region may appear swollen. Olecranon bursitis causes localised smooth swelling around the olecranon prominence (**134**): nodules within it may produce a lumpy contour.

Deformity
In particular, cubitus valgus or varus, and fixed extension (from in front); and posterior sub-luxation of the olecranon on the humerus (from behind).

Attitude
A capsular pattern of restriction usually affects flexion more than extension, with supination/pronation affected last: in the presence of syno-vitis or effusion the patient is therefore most comfortable with the elbow positioned in flexion (about 45–70°).

Inspection during movement

Ask the patient to bend up the elbow, assessing active flexion and extension for restriction and presence of stress pain. Then ask the patient to supinate and pronate the hands with the elbows tucked into the side at 90° flexion (**135**). If proximal or distal radioulnar (or humeroradial) joints are compromised, these movements may be painful and/or reduced: the patient often under-takes a trick manoeuvre, adducting the elbow across the abdomen to rotate the ulnar and thus increase supination (**136**).

Palpation

1 From behind
Stand behind the patient with their shoulder extended and elbow pointing backwards in mild flexion. Feel for:

Increased warmth
Pass the back of the hand over the distal upper arm, elbow, and forearm to detect increased warmth over the para-olecranon grooves and olecranon bursa.

Swelling, tenderness
Synovitis produces palpable soft-tissue swelling in the para-olecranon grooves: firm palpation at these sites may produce capsular tenderness (**137**).

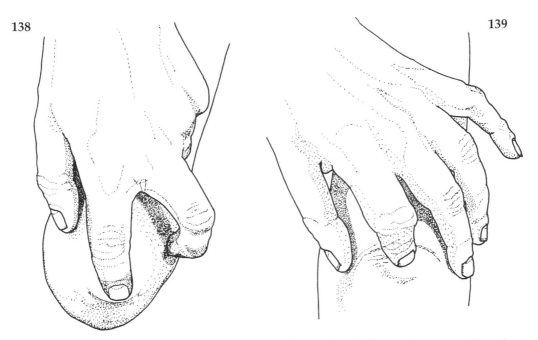

138, 139 Normal triangle sign: (**138**) in flexion, the examiner's fingers form an equilateral triangle; (**139**) in extension, the examiner's fingers form a straight line.

Feel for swelling of olecranon bursitis with the elbow extended: as the arm goes into flexion the bursa becomes more tense and prominent. A balloon sign will confirm a moderate-to-large fluid collection. Palpate for nodules along the extensor forearm border.

Deformity
The landmarks of the medial and lateral epicondyles are easily felt. Place a thumb and two fingers of one hand over the olecranon, medial epicondyle, and lateral epicondyle. In extension the three fingers form a straight line, in flexion they form an equilateral triangle (**138, 139**). Loss of such symmetry on flexion implies loss of height at the elbow due to cartilage and bone attrition ('triangle sign').

Crepitus
Place a finger in each para-olecranon groove to feel for crepitus from the humeroulnar and humeroradial joint while the patient flexes or extends.

Periarticular structures
On the medial side feel for the *ulnar nerve* below the epicondyle for thickening and disproportionate tenderness: this is the most common site for ulnar nerve entrapment. The medial supracondylar *lymph nodes* may be palpable if enlarged.

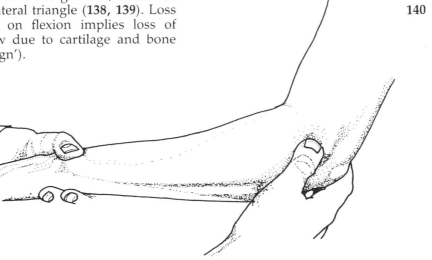

140 Palpation during pronation/supination.

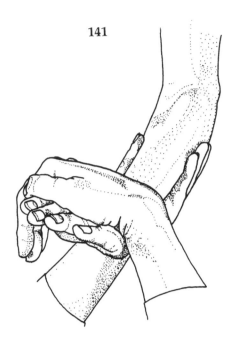

141 Resisted active wrist extension for lateral epicondylitis.

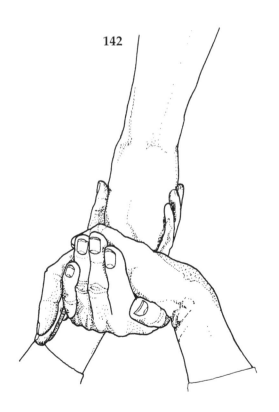

142 Resisted active wrist flexion for medial epicondylitis.

2 From in front
Increased warmth
Again use the back of the hand to feel for increased warmth over the radial head region.

Swelling
Palpate over the radial head for the soft-tissue swelling of synovitis. Occasionally, palpable anterior synovial extensions may almost fill the cubital fossa (predisposing to partial radial nerve palsy from pressure on the posterior interosseous nerve).

Proximal radioulnar joint (tenderness, laxity, crepitus, passive movement)
Pressure over the radial head may produce capsular/joint-line tenderness and, if there is associated joint damage and annular ligament laxity, excessive movement of the radial head with crepitus. Keeping the thumb over the radial head region, passively supinate and pronate with the other hand (the thumb is placed over the ulnar styloid region, **140**) to detect crepitus (both joints), assess range of passive movement, and enquire concerning pain.

Passive movement humeroulnar joint
Assess the range of passive flexion and extension (looking for restriction ± stress pain) and compare with active movements: similar restriction suggests synovitis; a greater passive range favours a neuromuscular rather than joint cause.

Epicondylar tenderness, resisted active movements
For tennis elbow, palpate for tenderness over the common extensor origin at the lateral epicondyle: in some cases tenderness is more distal, occurring over the radial head region. Confirmation is by resisted active wrist extension, which reproduces the pain (**141**). For golfer's elbow, palpate for tenderness over the medial epicondyle at the insertion of the wrist flexor/pronator group (pronator teres, flexor carpi radialis, palmaris longus, flexor carpi ulnaris). Resisted active wrist flexion with the hand supinated reproduces the pain (**142**).

ADDITIONAL TESTS

Collateral ligament stability

This may be tested by flexing the patient's elbow to about 20–30° and then holding the elbow in one hand while applying a progressive varus force (testing the lateral ligament) followed by a valgus force (medial ligament) on the distal forearm (**143**), noting any pain or increased lateral movement.

Tests for nerve entrapment at elbow

The ulnar is affected more commonly than median or radial nerves. Helpful tests include:

Tinel's sign
Light percussion over the ulnar nerve as it travels through the medial para-olecranon groove produces tingling in an ulnar distribution in the forearm/hand distal to the point of compression (**144**).

Elbow flexion test
The patient holds the elbow in full flexion for 5 min. Tingling in an ulnar distribution again suggests a cubital tunnel syndrome.

143

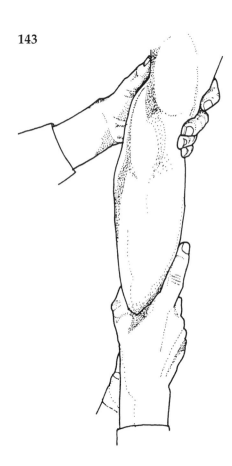

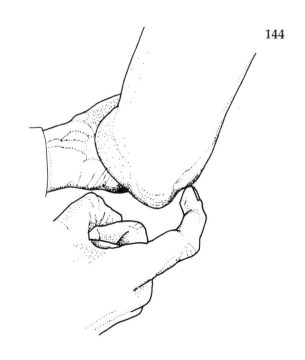

144

143 Testing collateral ligament stability.

144 Tinel's sign.

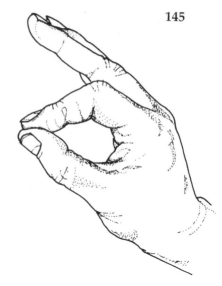

Pinch grip test

The patient attempts to oppose the tips of the index finger and thumb. If the normal tip-to-tip pinch is replaced by a pulp-to-pulp pinch (**145**), reflecting impairment of index finger and thumb flexors, entrapment of the anterior interosseus nerve, as it passes between the two heads of the pronator teres, is suggested (*'anterior interosseous nerve syndrome'*). If the median nerve is compressed just prior to the anterior interosseous division, the flexor carpi radialis, palmaris longus and flexor digitorum muscles are also weak (*'pronator teres syndrome'*). In both cases there is sensory impairment in a median nerve distribution. Rarely, the median nerve is compressed as it passes (± the brachial artery) beneath the ligament of Struthers, an anomalous band in 1% of people that runs from a spur on the humerus to the medial epicondyle; in this case (*'humerus supracondylar process syndrome'*) the pronator teres is also involved (± vascular, as well as neurological, symptoms).

145   Pinch grip test.

SUMMARY OF ELBOW EXAMINATION

(1) Inspection at rest
    skin changes
    swelling (synovitis, bursitis, nodules)
    deformity (valgus, varus, posterior subluxation)
    attitude
(2) Inspection during movement
    flexion/extension
    supination/pronation
(3) Palpation from behind
    warmth
    para-olecranon grooves
        swelling
        tenderness
        crepitus
        deformity (triangle sign)
        palpable ulnar nerve, enlarged nodes
    olecranon region (bursa, nodules)
(4) Palpation from in front
    warmth
    swelling
    radial head (proximal radioulnar joint)
        tenderness
        laxity
        crepitus
    passive movements
        supination/pronation
        flexion/extension
    peri-epicondylar tenderness
    resisted active wrist extension (tennis elbow)
    resisted active wrist flexion (golfer's elbow)

5 Shoulder

The shoulder girdle comprises three joints (sterno-clavicular, acromioclavicular, and glenohumeral) and one articulation (scapulothoracic).

The *sternoclavicular joint* (SCJ) is a saddle-shaped synovial joint that connects the medial clavicle, manubrium sternum, and cartilage of the first rib (**146**). It is divided into two cavities by a fibrocartilage disc. The capsule is strengthened by the sternoclavicular (anterior and posterior) and interclavicular ligaments; the costoclavicular ligament binds the undersurface of the clavicle to the first rib.

The *acromioclavicular joint* (ACJ) is a plane syno-vial joint, angled to allow the clavicle to slide over the acromion (**147, 148**); a disc is variably present. Stability is due to the coracoclavicular ligament (comprising lateral 'trapezoid' and medial 'conoid' portions) and the acromioclavicular ligament. The joint has sensory branches to the suprascapular and long thoracic nerves.

The *glenohumeral joint* is a multiaxial, spheroidal synovial joint (**149**). Its range of movement, greater than that of any other joint, is permitted at the expense of stability. The glenoid fossa, though widened by the fibrocartilaginous labrum, is shallow, the capsule is lax and thin, and there are no strong traversing ligaments. Stability primarily depends on the muscles and conjoining tendons of the rotator cuff (**150, 151**). Supraspinatus, infra-spinatus and teres minor arise posteriorly on the scapula and insert into the greater tuberosity; subscapularis arises anteriorly on the scapula and inserts into the lesser tuberosity. The deltoid and the rotator cuff form a mechanical couple: the rotators stabilise the humerus and cause the head to 'drop down' into the lower, wider part of the glenoid cavity, converting the deltoid's upward pull into a powerful abducting force.

The joint is protected superiorly by an 'arch' formed by the coracoid process, the acromion, and the coracoacromial ligament. The lax capsule has a deep inferior fold and two openings (see **148**); one allows the long head of the biceps tendon to enter the bicipital groove (taking an extension of the synovium with it as its sheath: **152**), the other permits an outpouching of the synovium to act as a bursa for the subscapularis.

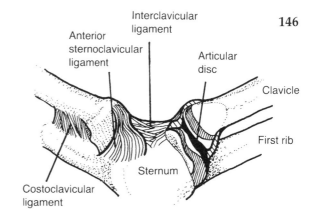

146

146   The sternoclavicular joint.

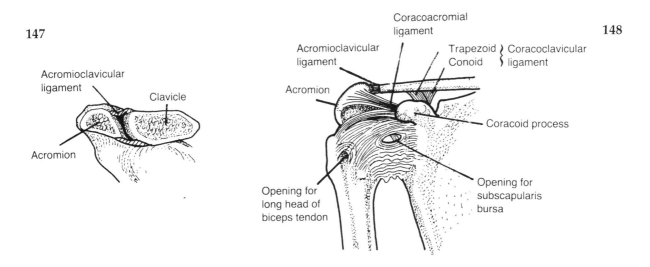

147

148

147, 148   The acromioclavicular joint, ligaments and glenohumeral capsule.

149

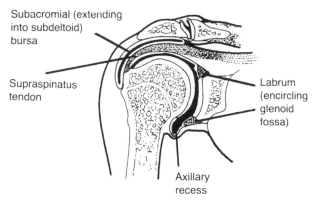

Subacromial (extending into subdeltoid) bursa

Supraspinatus tendon

Labrum (encircling glenoid fossa)

Axillary recess

149 The glenohumeral joint (in section).

A large subacromial bursa permits smooth movement between the rotator cuff and the undersurface of the acromion: it extends laterally into the subdeltoid bursa. The subacromial bursa communicates with the joint cavity in some normal individuals: since the supraspinatus tendon forms the floor of the bursa and the roof of the capsule, any tear of the tendon/cuff is likely to lead to communication between the two. The subcoracoid bursa, between the coracoid and the capsule, may be separate or communicate with the subacromial bursa. The suprascapular nerve supplies the superior and posterior parts of the joint and capsule and most of the rotator cuff; the axillary nerve supplies the anterior aspect of the joint and capsule.

150 Subscapularis

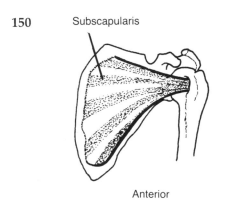

Anterior

151 Supraspinatus

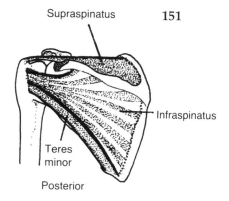

Infraspinatus

Teres minor

Posterior

150, 151 Rotator cuff muscles.

152

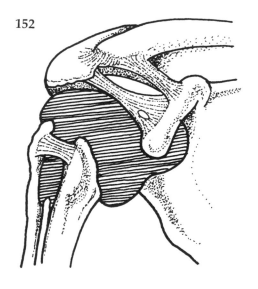

152 Synovial limits, and extension around the biceps tendon (long head) in the bicipital groove.

The SCJ is commonly affected by major arthropathies (e.g. rheumatoid, osteoarthritis, seronegative spondyloarthropathy), and is an occasional site for sepsis, particularly in the immunocompromised. Although it is common to find abnormal signs at the SCJ, it is an uncommon site for symptoms. The ACJ is also often involved in major arthropathies (particularly osteoarthritis); unlike the SCJ, it is a common source of symptoms. The glenohumeral joint may be involved in inflammatory arthropathy (e.g. rheumatoid, seronegative spondyloarthropathies): though an uncommon site for 'primary' osteoarthritis it is often involved in the subset of pyrophosphate arthropathy in the elderly. Rotator cuff injuries are exceedingly common, and the cuff and bursae can be directly involved in inflammatory conditions. Because of its close relationships, subacromial bursitis can result from pathology relating to the rotator cuff, ACJ, or the glenohumeral joint.

The scapulothoracic articulation is of little rheumatological interest. It is a common site of painless, reproducible grating, or 'clonking': such noises are, in general, abolished by moving the scapula laterally and merely reflect movement over uneven surfaces.

SYMPTOMS

SCJ pain is usually well localised, with little radiation (153). The ACJ derives from C4 and produces pain close to its origin, with some radiation to the shoulder tip but no significant radiation to the arm. All glenohumeral joint structures, including the rotator cuff and the subacromial bursa, develop from the C5 sclerotome and produce pain maximal at the outer aspect of the upper arm close to the deltoid insertion; if severe, pain may radiate down the radial aspect of the forearm to the elbow (rarely to the wrist) and upwards to the shoulder (rarely to the neck). Such pain will be worsened by shoulder movements. Tendinitis of the long head of biceps also produces upper arm pain (C5/6).

Pain over the superior aspect of the shoulder and the C4/5 distribution (154) may also be referred from the neck: such pain may involve the whole length of the arm (± the hand), be worsened by neck movements (and only the extremes of shoulder movements), and be accompanied by sensory or motor impairment in the limb. Radiation of pain into the arm associated with numbness, or paraesthesia, suggests compressive neuropathy (e.g. thoracic outlet syndrome, suprascapular or axillary nerve entrapment). Lesions involving or close to the diaphragm may cause pain referred to the shoulder tip region, unrelated to shoulder movement. Myocardial pain may produce variable aching and pain down the arm.

Differentiation between glenohumeral-joint and rotator-cuff disease is often suggested by the history (*Table 8*). A typical rotator-cuff patient has often performed unaccustomed exercise with the involved arm (e.g. decorating the ceiling): the patient usually notices nothing at the time, but the following day complains of upper arm aching as a single regional pain syndrome. Pain is non-progressive and is usually noted only during one or two movements of the arm (e.g. reaching up to a shelf): it is generally more an inconvenience than a major problem, and uncommonly interferes with sleep. Conversely, though acute monoarthritis of the glenohumeral joint can occur, arthritis at this site is usually part of an oligo- or polyarthritis that produces multiple regional pain problems. Pain is often insidious in onset without an obvious provoking event: it is variable but usually progressive, often keeps the patient awake, affects several (eventually all) shoulder movements, and tends to interfere greatly with simple activities of daily living. Acute subacromial or subdeltoid bursitis is often characterised by its speed of onset, the patient being unable to abduct the arm within just a few days.

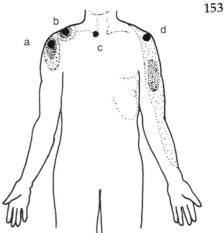

153 Pain patterns around the shoulder: (a) bicipital tendinitis; (b) acromioclavicular joint; (c) sternoclavicular joint; (d) glenohumeral joint/rotator cuff/subacromial bursitis.

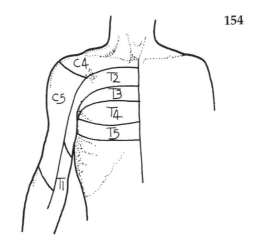

154 Dermatomes around the shoulder.

Table 8. Comparison between typical symptoms arising from rotator cuff lesions and glenohumeral arthritis.

	Rotator cuff	Glenohumeral arthritis
Pain: onset	Acute	Insidious
progression	Non-progressive	Variable, progressive
Movements affected	Few	Many
Provoking factor	Often apparent	Absent
Localised problem	Usually	Uncommonly
Severity	+ +	+ + + +

INSPECTION AT REST

Get the patient standing or seated on a chair or the side of the couch/bed, to permit inspection from in front and from behind.

Inspection from in front

Look at the SCJ region where the jugular notch above the manubrium is clearly evident (**155**). Look for erythema and swelling overlying the medial end of the clavicle: fluid from the joint will appear as a smooth rounded swelling; irregular swelling is more likely to be osteophyte. If the SCJ is subluxed the medial end of the clavicle comes anteriorly, medially, and inferiorly across the sternum, appearing more prominent than usual (comparison between the two sides is helpful if unilateral). Look along the clavicle for irregularity and bony swelling (e.g. from an old fracture, Paget's, or a primary or secondary tumour).

The site of the ACJ may be apparent due to prominence of the lateral end of the clavicle, but in many subjects this is a flat joint with no surface landmark. Inspection over the approximate area proximal to the shoulder tip, however, may show erythema or swelling (fluid at this site is rare and swelling usually reflects osteophyte).

Inspect muscle bulk. All individuals, whatever their age, should have a convex, full deltoid. Large glenohumeral effusions are uncommon but if present may push anteromedially and present as a swelling which fills the usual triangular depression bordered superiorly by the lateral end of the clavicle, laterally by the medial curve of the deltoid, and inferiorly by pectoralis (**156**). A large subdeltoid bursa may cause undue prominence of the deltoid contour. The typical attitude of a patient with glenohumeral arthropathy is for the shoulder to be held in internal rotation and adduction, with the hand folded across the abdomen as if in a sling: this is the most comfortable position for minimising intra-articular hypertension (conversely, when the examiner comes to palpation, the opposite movements — external rotation and abduction — are the earliest and most severely involved, in terms of pain and restriction).

Inspection from behind

Now go behind the patient and again inspect for muscle bulk on the two sides, looking particularly at the supraspinatus and the infraspinatus muscles, but also comparing the trapezius and rhomboid muscle bulk. Glenohumeral lesions commonly cause generalised wasting of shoulder girdle muscles. Isolated wasting, e.g. of supraspinatus muscle, suggests a local periarticular lesion. Occasionally, a congenitally underdeveloped, elevated scapula may be noted (Sprengel's deformity).

155

Prominence of clavicle

Triangular depression

SCJ

ACJ

Convex deltoid

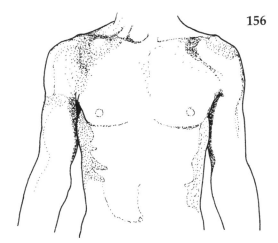

156

155 Normal surface landmarks (anterior view).

156 Swelling due to right glenohumeral joint effusion.

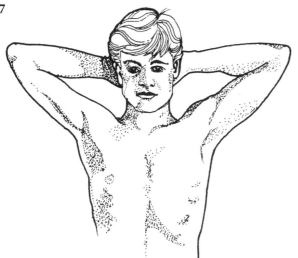

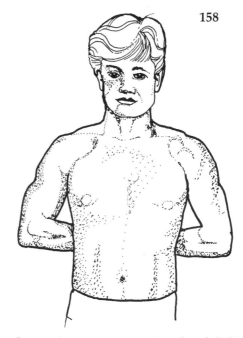

157 Composite movement testing: 'hands behind the head'.

158 Composite movement testing: 'hands behind the back'.

INSPECTION DURING MOVEMENT

All individual glenohumeral movements can be examined in turn, comparing one side with the other; but to quickly screen for joint and rotator cuff problems ask the patient to perform two composite active movements (**157, 158**):

- Place the hands round behind the neck (testing abduction, external rotation, and flexion of the glenohumeral joint and the supraspinatus, infraspinatus, and teres minor muscles).
- Take the hands down and round behind the back (testing internal rotation, abduction and extension of the glenohumeral joint, and principally, the subscapularis muscle).

If the patient is able to perform both movements without any problem the glenohumeral and rotator cuff apparatus are probably normal.

However, if the patient has pain or difficulty with these actions, look for a painful arc. For this, ask the patient to raise the arm slowly through 180° towards the ceiling, and then slowly to lower it again. This is a composite movement (**159**), the initial 90° representing glenohumeral abduction, the next 70° being principally scapula rotation, and the final 20° being further glenohumeral movement. During the latter-half of this composite movement the SCJ and ACJ are also moving, and many people also tend to rotate their arm. Two principal patterns of painful arc may be observed: painful middle arc and superior painful arc.

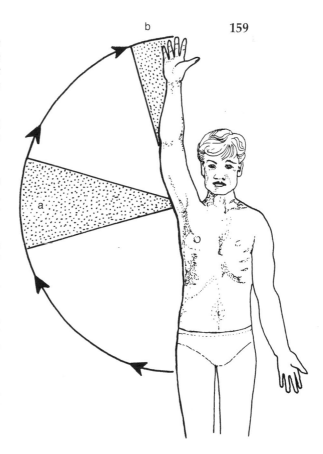

159 Painful arc patterns: (a) middle arc (supraspinatus/subacromial bursitis); (b) superior arc (ACJ).

1 Painful middle arc

The patient experiences pain when the hand gets within the central 30° or so of the painful arc (i.e. around the end of initial glenohumeral abduction). In this situation the greater tuberosity of the humerus rises relative to the acromion and can squeeze the intervening structures (supraspinatus tendon and subacromial bursa). As the arm is further elevated the greater tuberosity drops relative to the acromion and relieves the pressure. This arc is characteristic of a supraspinatus lesion or subacromial bursitis. Supination of the hand may decrease impingement of the humerus on the acromion and reduce or eliminate the pain in the middle arc.

2 Superior painful arc

Pain occurs at the top 20–30° of the arc. This is when there is maximal stress on the ACJ, suggesting a lesion of that joint.

Occasionally, patients with supraspinatus lesions have no painful arc on moving their arm upwards, but on slowly lowering the arm they experience a painful catching sensation in the middle-arc range, which causes them to quickly drop the arm to their side. The patient should therefore be asked to take the arm slowly up *and* down.

PALPATION

Palpation is best conducted from behind. With the patient seated, the standing examiner is in an ideal position. A typical procedure is as follows:

To palpate the SCJ, identify the manubrial notch, then take the fingers laterally to the medial end of the clavicle. Having found the approximate position ask the patient to move the joint by shrugging the shoulders upwards (**160**). This will allow the examiner to:

- Confirm the position of the joint.
- Feel for crepitus.
- Feel for subluxation (shrugging exaggerates subluxation and the examiner may feel the medial end of the clavicle push his fingers anteriorly, inferiorly, and medially across the front of the manubrium).

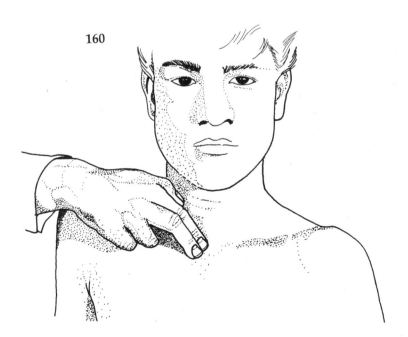

160

160 Palpation of SCJ as patient shrugs shoulders.

Having found the SCJ, press firmly for joint tenderness. Palpate for swelling to determine whether it is soft or bony (bony osteophyte is the most common cause of swelling). If the swelling is soft, look for a balloon sign by placing two fingers of one hand at opposite limits of the swelling and pressing with the other hand over its centre. Pass the back of the hand over the joint and with the same sweep continue over the clavicle and the ACJ to determine increased temperature at each site. Palpate along the clavicle for any obvious localised tenderness and then come to the ACJ.

The site of the ACJ may be visible if the distal end of the clavicle is prominent. However, if unsure, feel the outermost bony contour at the shoulder tip (i.e. the coracoid as it slopes posteriorly) and palpate approximately two fingers' breadth in from that site (this approximates to the joint line in adults). With the fingers in the approximate joint position ask the patient to move the joint by shrugging the shoulder or abducting the arm. This allows the examiner to:

- Localise the correct joint site.
- Feel for crepitus.

Having found the joint line, press on it for tenderness (161) and palpate for soft or bony swelling (the latter, resulting from osteophyte, is again most common). If the swelling is soft, look for a balloon sign (rarely present). If the ACJ appears to be the main problem, forced adduction of the arm across the front of the patient's chest stresses the joint and may reproduce the pain (this movement is not painful in glenohumeral disease).

The glenohumeral joint is well protected from the examiner's hands by the partially encircling rotator cuff, the acromion superiorly, and the overlying deltoid. The anterior part of the joint is the most accessible for palpation. Start by palpating the anterior triangular region just inferior to the clavicle at the medial border of the deltoid: if there is any soft-tissue fullness (suggesting a glenohumeral effusion) press firmly and then release to see if fluid refills the swelling. Move the palpating finger laterally from this position to identify the forward-pointing coracoid process. Taking the finger further laterally (between the coracoid process medially and the humeral head laterally: 162) push firmly upwards and backwards to elicit any anterior joint-line/capsular tenderness (often marked in glenohumeral arthritis and 'capsulitis').

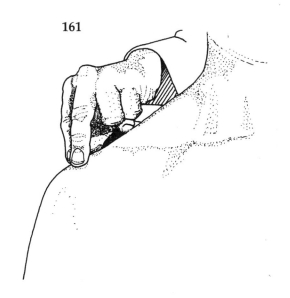

161 Palpation of ACJ.

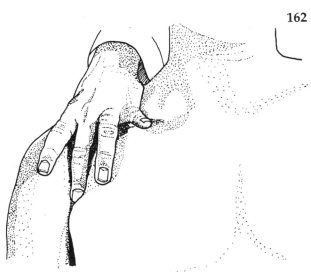

162 Palpation for anterior glenohumeral joint-line tenderness.

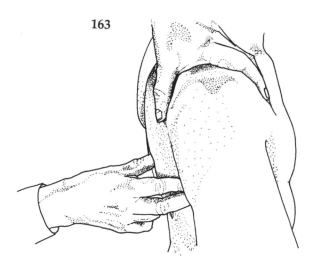

163 Position of hands while testing active abduction at the glenohumeral joint.

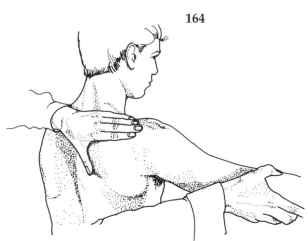

164 Passive abduction at the glenohumeral joint.

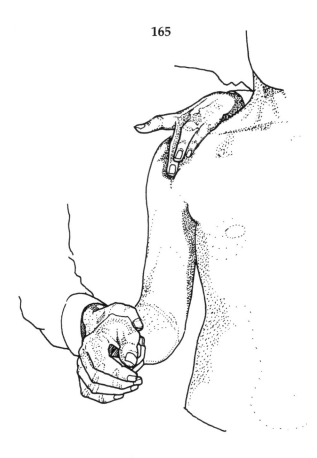

165 Palpating for tenderness over the biceps tendon.

Keep the fingers over the anterior joint line to feel for crepitus while the glenohumeral joint is now moved. Since abduction and external rotation are the movements affected earliest and maximally by glenohumeral disease they are good screening movements to test. First, locate the blade of the scapula and place the thumb and finger either side of its lower limit so that any scapula movement can be identified. With one hand palpating for crepitus over the anterior joint line and the other holding onto the scapula (**163**), ask the patient to slowly take the arm out in abduction and assess the range of movement (normally 80–90°). If there is glenohumeral restriction the examiner will feel the scapular move early before the arm has got to 90°: the patient often performs a trick manoeuvre, with hunching of the shoulder up towards the ear. If active abduction is painful, determine whether this is in a stress–pain pattern (progressive pain towards the limit of restricted abduction). If pain or restriction of active abduction is present, rest one hand on top of the spine of the scapula (to assess scapula movement) and passively abduct the arm with the other hand to determine the extent of passive glenohumeral abduction (**164**). In glenohumeral/capsular disease, active and passive findings will be similar for both pain and degree of restriction. If, however, passive movement is far greater and less painful than active movement, a muscle/tendon (or nerve) lesion is more likely.

166

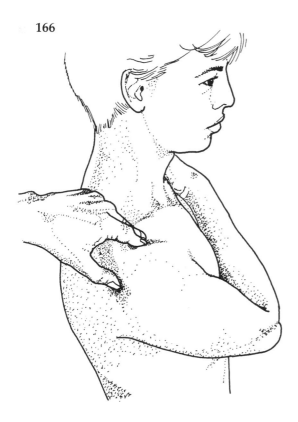

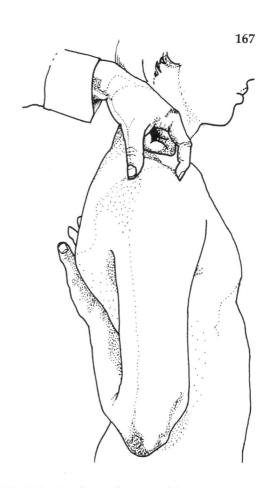

167

166 Palpation for tenderness of the posterior aspect of the rotator cuff.

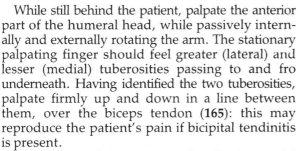

While still behind the patient, palpate the anterior part of the humeral head, while passively internally and externally rotating the arm. The stationary palpating finger should feel greater (lateral) and lesser (medial) tuberosities passing to and fro underneath. Having identified the two tuberosities, palpate firmly up and down in a line between them, over the biceps tendon (**165**): this may reproduce the patient's pain if bicipital tendinitis is present.

Tenderness of the rotator cuff and subacromial bursa can also be sought while the examiner stands behind the patient. The cuff is protected beneath the acromion while the patient's arm is by the side. If the patient places the hand onto the opposite shoulder, however, this produces posterior rotation of the humeral head and will partly bring the rotator cuff from underneath the protective cover of the acromion. Palpation just below the posterior aspect of the acromion may

167 Palpation for tenderness of the anterior aspect of the rotator cuff.

then elicit tenderness of the posterior part of the rotator cuff (**166**). Similarly, if the patient places the hand round behind the back, this causes anterior movement of the humeral head and brings the anterior part of the cuff from beneath the acromion. Palpation just in front of the acromion will then elicit tenderness of the anterior part of the cuff (**167**). Palpation below the lateral part of the acromion may occasionally produce tenderness in subacromial/subdeltoid bursitis. Palpation directly over the supraspinatus and infraspinatus may produce tenderness in lesions of these muscles.

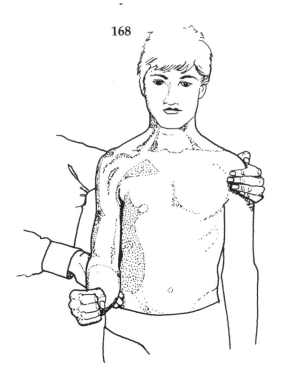

168

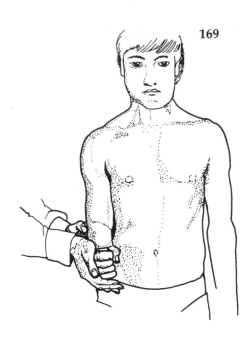

169

168 Resisted active abduction.

169 Resisted active external rotation.

RESISTED ACTIVE MOVEMENTS

Resisted active movements are used to detect rotator cuff lesions. Sit alongside the patient and place the patient's elbow at their side with the elbow at 90° and the hand pointing forwards with clenched fist and thumb upwards. The following movements are then tested:

- *Resisted active abduction.* Abduction is a strong movement and the examiner should place his arm around the patient and hold onto the other shoulder while the patient is asked to push their elbow outwards against the examiner's hand (**168**). Supraspinatus initiates abduction and with lesions of the muscle or tendon this attempted movement will reproduce pain in the upper arm (away from the examiner's restraining hand). If the patient had a painful middle arc and resisted active abduction reproduces pain then a supraspinatus lesion is the likely cause of pain. If, however, they have a painful middle arc and resisted active abduction is pain-free then the likely problem is subacromial bursitis (resisted active abduction does nothing to the subacromial bursa).

- *Resisted active external rotation.* Steady the patient's elbow at their side with one hand (to prevent any abduction) and ask the patient to push the hand outwards against the examiner's other restraining hand (**169**). Pain experienced in the upper arm suggests an infraspinatus/teres minor lesion.
- *Resisted internal rotation.* Again, steady the patient's elbow at their side and ask them to push the hand inwards against the examiner's restraining other hand (**170**). Pain experienced in the upper arm suggests a subscapularis muscle/tendon lesion.

Weakness of any of these movements may result from pain, partial or complete tears of the cuff, or from neurological abnormality (if power is restored following injection of a local anaesthetic into the subacromial space, pain inhibition rather than rupture is implied).

Bicipital tendinitis is also tested by resisted active movement (**171**). With the patient's arm in the same position as for rotator cuff testing, hold onto the patient's clenched fist with both hands

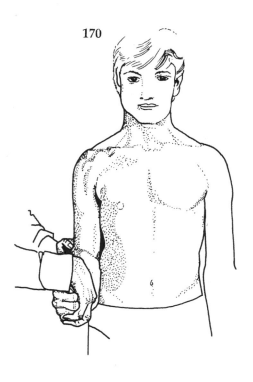

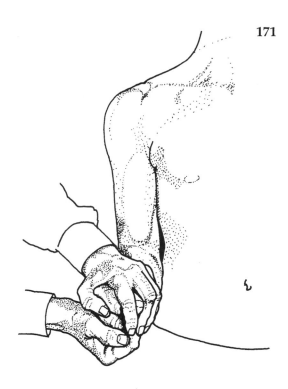

170 Resisted active internal rotation.

171 Resisted supination for bicipital tendinitis.

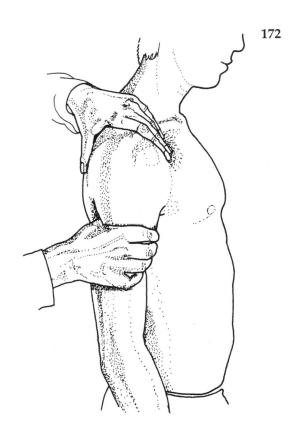

and ask the patient to turn the wrist outwards in supination. This is a very strong movement and the examiner can observe the biceps tensing up: upper arm pain will be reproduced with bicipital tendinitis. If the patient has ruptured the tendon of the long head of biceps, the muscle bulge produced by this manoeuvre will be predominantly in the distal part of the upper arm, producing a larger, more localised, swelling than usual.

TESTS FOR GLENOHUMERAL INSTABILITY

These are particularly important in the younger patient with a history suggestive of subluxation/ dislocation (sometimes as part of generalised hypermobility). Stability should be tested in anterior, posterior, and inferior directions.

With the patient standing, and the arm hanging relaxed by their side, fix the scapula and shoulder girdle from behind with one hand while gripping the top of the humerus with the other (**172**): move

172 Testing for anterior and posterior instability.

the humeral head backwards and forwards in the glenoid fossa, noting the degree of movement and any palpable clicks which may signify labral pathology. Next, position the patient with their shoulder abducted to 90° and the elbow flexed (**173**). Gently, passively extend and externally rotate the glenohumeral joint: a positive test for anterior instability is when the patient experiences apprehension as an external rotation force is applied.

A more controlled method involves the patient lying supine, with the shoulder at the edge of the couch. Support the arm with one hand while fixing the scapula/girdle firmly with the other: move the humeral head anteriorly, posteriorly, and inferiorly using direct pressure. Pain may be reproduced at the limits of movement. If there is significant inferior subluxation a distinct gap may be felt between the humerus and the acromion. As in the apprehension test, position the arm in abduction and external rotation until the patient experiences discomfort: backward pressure on the upper humerus (i.e. anterior glenohumeral support) may now relieve the patient's pain and permit further passive external rotation. If the stabilising force to the upper arm is then removed, the patient may again experience pain if anterior instability is present. Flexion of the arm in this position, with gentle axial pressure, can be used to demonstrate posterior subluxation.

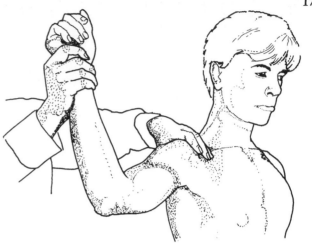

173 'Apprehension' test.

SUMMARY OF SHOULDER EXAMINATION

(1) Inspection at rest
    from in front (skin changes, swelling, wasting, attitude)
    from behind (wasting, Sprengel's deformity)
(2) Inspection during movement
    'hands behind head', 'hands behind back'
    painful arc
(3) Palpation
    SCJ (crepitus, subluxation, tenderness, swelling, warmth)
    ACJ (crepitus, tenderness, swelling, warmth)
    glenohumeral joint:
        effusion
        anterior joint-line/capsular tenderness
        active abduction (restriction, pain, crepitus)
        passive abduction (restriction, pain)
    periarticular tenderness (biceps tendon, rotator cuff, muscles, bursae)
(4) Resisted active movements (weakness, pain)
    abduction (supraspinatus)
    external rotation (infraspinatus, teres minor)
    internal rotation (subscapularis)
    wrist supination (biceps)

6 Spine and Sacroiliac Joints

The unique structure of the vertebral column serves to protect the spinal cord, accompanying vessels, and viscera, and to allow controlled movement of the back, neck and head. The normal balanced spinal curves (cervical and lumbar lordosis, thoracic and sacral kyphosis; **174**) help maintain an upright posture with minimal muscular effort and, together with the resilience of the intervertebral discs, facilitate impact loading through the spine.

The *vertebrae* from C3 to L5 have a common pattern of an anterior vertebral body and a posterior neural arch (**175–177**). The arch comprises three processes, two lateral (transverse) and one posterior (spinous), that are primarily adapted for muscle attachment, and a synovial facet or *apophyseal joints* above and below, for articulation with adjacent arches. The bodies and their separating discs are the main weight-bearing portions, body size increasing from C2 to the first sacral

174

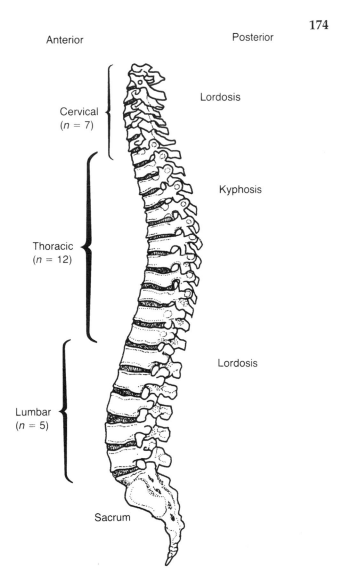

Anterior Posterior

Lordosis

Cervical (*n* = 7)

Kyphosis

Thoracic (*n* = 12)

Lordosis

Lumbar (*n* = 5)

Sacrum

174 Spinal vertebrae and curvatures.

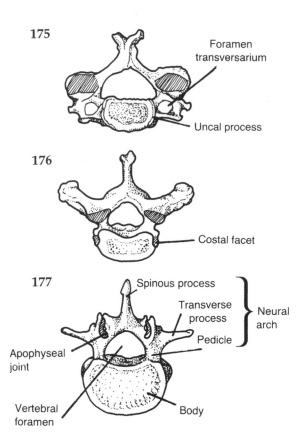

175

Foramen transversarium

Uncal process

176

Costal facet

177

Spinous process

Transverse process

Neural arch

Pedicle

Apophyseal joint

Vertebral foramen

Body

175–177 Vertebral configuration at different levels: (175) cervical; (176) thoracic; (177) lumbar.

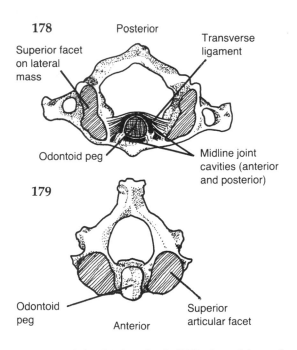

178

Posterior

Superior facet on lateral mass

Transverse ligament

Odontoid peg

Midline joint cavities (anterior and posterior)

179

Odontoid peg

Anterior

Superior articular facet

178,179 Atlas (178) and axis (179) viewed from above.

segment, then decreasing down to the coccyx as body weight transmits to the pelvis. The sliding apophyseal joints help stabilise the vertebrae, particularly limiting anterior displacement: varying alignment of their articular surfaces largely determines the extent and type of movement at different regions. Differences between levels are superimposed on this basic pattern:

- *Cervical vertebrae* have foramina in the transverse processes for vertebral arteries, and superolateral ridges (uncal processes) for the joints of Luschka (these increase lateral stability while facilitating free motion between vertebrae).
- *Thoracic vertebrae* have long transverse processes directed posteriorly; articular facets for ribs occur on their tips and on the posterior corners of the bodies.
- *Lumbar vertebrae* have facet joints orientated in the saggital plane.

The *atlas* (C1) and the *axis* (C2) are unique (**178, 179**), the axis having the odontoid peg, and the atlas being a ring that receives the odontoid peg anteriorly, held in place by the transverse ligament. No disc exists between the atlas and the axis (or occiput and atlas), the axis articulating with the atlas through midline and paired lateral synovial joints. The *midline joint* has two synovial cavities that extend between the peg and anterior arch of the atlas, and between the peg and transverse ligament: synovitis here may damage the peg and ligament, leading to C1/C2 instability and cord damage.

Intervertebral discs (IVDs) are complex symphyses comprising about 25% of the total height of the spine. Each consists of two zones (**180, 181**):

- The outermost fibrocartilaginous *annulus fibrosus*, with concentrically arranged fibres (kept under tension by the nucleus), firm attachment to the vertebral bodies, and innervation to its outer layer. The interwoven concentric fibre arrangement affords great tensile strength while facilitating torsional movements.
- The central mucoid *nucleus pulposus*, containing a high proportion of water, permitting shape (but not volume) change in response to compressive force. Loss of spinal height with age largely results from decrease in water content of the nucleus (from about 90% in youth to 65% in old age: associated decrease in turgor slackens tension in the annulus, predisposing to tears).

IVD height (and movement between vertebrae) is greatest in the cervical and lumbar regions, and their anteroposterior asymmetry largely determines the normal spinal curves. Posture has a profound effect on intra-disc pressure, particularly at the lumbosacral junction where forward flexion associates with the highest increase. The lumbosacral junction is the point of transition between movable and immovable parts of the spine: the spine can act as a lever on the pelvis at this point (this, together with the marked angulation between L4, L5, and S1, makes it a common site for spondylolisthesis). Particularly vulnerable to mechanical stress, the lumbosacral region is also a common site for congenital anomalies of the vertebrae and abnormalities of the IVDs.

The spine is stabilised by numerous strong ligaments (**182**). The *posterior* and *anterior longitudinal ligaments* run the length of the spine attaching to discs (particularly the posterior ligament) and vertebral bodies (especially the stronger anterior ligament): they act to restrict flexion and extension and protect the discs. There are also ligaments between adjacent vertebral arches (ligamenta flava), transverse processes (intertransverse ligaments) and spinous processes (interspinous and supraspinous ligaments).

The large superficial *muscles* of the back (trapezius, latissimus dorsi) largely cover the deeper layers of intrinsic muscles within the lumbodorsal fascia. The numerous deep longitudinal muscles join adjacent segments and span several segments. The longest and strongest extensors are the *erector spinae* (sacrospinalis), which run either side of the spinous processes, from the sacrum to the skull; they are most developed in the lumbar region. The supra and infra hyoid muscles assist in neck flexion; the pectoralis minor and major assist thoracic flexion; and most lumbar flexion is by the paired rectus abdominae, assisted by muscles attached to the anterior vertebrae (quadratus lumborum, iliopsoas). Lateral flexion and rotation is achieved by the oblique abdominal muscles. The neck has a complex system of musculature that enables fine movements to be accurately controlled.

Movement of occipital condyles on the atlas produces discrete nodding (about 30°), and the atlanto-axial joint permits discrete rotation (about 30°) of the head. Below the craniocervical junction, movement involves distortion of IVDs and sliding movements of the facet joints. Flexion and extension is mainly at the low cervical and low lumbar spine, lateral flexion is greatest in the neck, and rotation greatest in the lower thoracic spine.

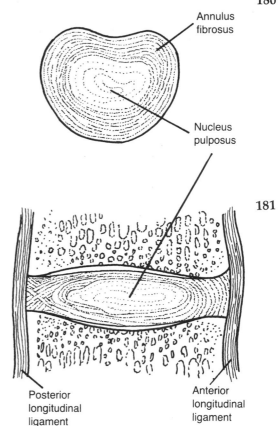

180, 181 Intervertebral disc structure: (**180**) disc viewed from above, showing concentric fibre arrangement; (**181**) saggital section.

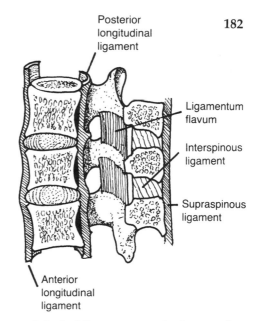

182 Principal ligaments attached to vertebrae.

The variable *sacroiliac joints* (SIJs) lie between the wedge-shaped sacrum and the medial aspect of each ilium (**183, 184**). Fibrocartilage covers the iliac side, and thicker hyaline cartilage the sacral side. The lower portion of each SIJ is aligned in an anteroposterior plane, but the upper portion is oblique, with the ilia extending beyond the lateral aspect of the sacrum posteriorly. Viewed from in front, the upper one-third (superior, posterior) is a fibrous joint (syndesmosis), while the lower two-thirds (anterior, inferior) is synovial. The bones are bound by ventral and dorsal interosseous, sacrotuberous, sacrospinous and iliolumbar ligaments and, except in pregnancy (and childhood), there is no movement.

Basic *neurological aspects* require consideration in respect of the spine. The narrow, rigid confines of the spinal canal and emerging foramina may cause problems relating to root or, less commonly, cord compression. The cervical cord is widest and most susceptible to compression; it is also vulnerable to damage by atlanto-axial subluxation. The lumbar cord ends opposite the L1/2 disc space, so lower lesions cause root syndromes only. *Nerve roots* are most vulnerable as they emerge from their dural sheaths, just after leaving the exit foramina: they lie in the immediate path of a prolapsing lateral disc. In the lumbar spine such prolapse compresses the *lower* emerging root. Cervical roots C1–C7 emerge over the top of their respective vertebra, but the C8 root emerges below C7 and above T1 (giving eight cervical roots but only seven vertebrae). Below T1 all roots emerge below their respective vertebrae. Movements and their root supplies are shown in **185** and **186**; dermatomes are shown in **187** and **188**.

Upright posture is still a relatively recent evolutionary development. As a result of high mechanical stresses through the spine (amplified by poor posture and muscle tone, and obesity), sprain injuries of ligaments, entheses, and muscles are particularly common. Apophyseal joint osteoarthritis and degenerative disc disease are also common, especially at the mobile, stressed lower cervical and lower lumbar regions: root

183

Iliolumbar ligament

Fibrous upper one-third

Ventral interosseous ligament

Synovial lower two-thirds

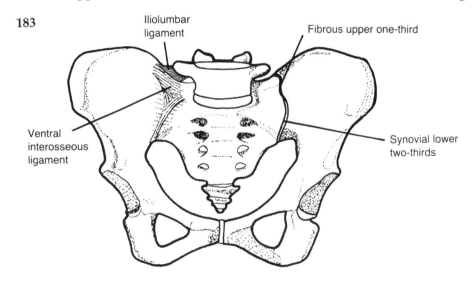

184

Dorsal sacroiliac ligament

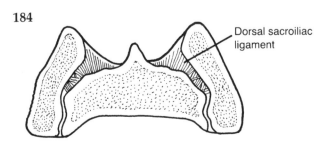

183, 184   The sacroiliac joints viewed from in front (**183**) and in transverse section (**184**).

syndromes, caused by pressure from extruded disc material or bony encroachment (particularly apophyseal joint osteophyte) also predominate here. Less commonly, spinal joints and entheses are target sites for inflammatory disease (especially, seronegative spondyloarthropathy), and bone involvement by malignancy or sepsis may also occur.

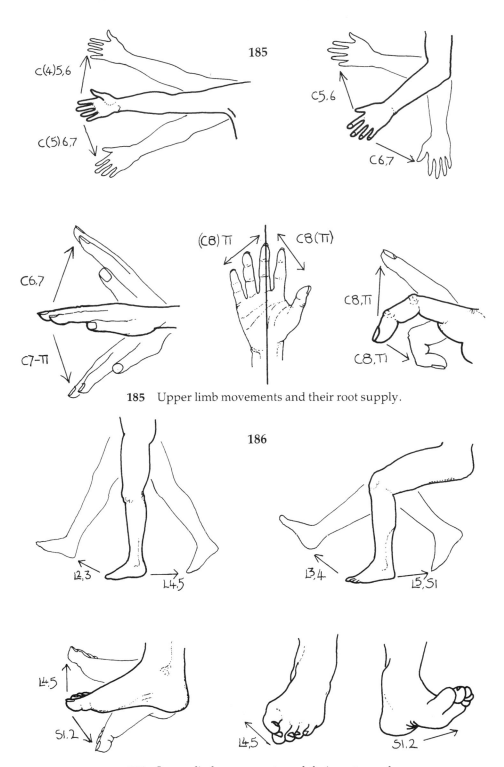

185 Upper limb movements and their root supply.

186 Lower limb movements and their root supply.

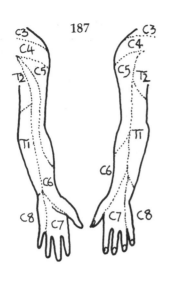

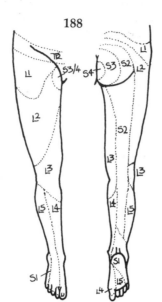

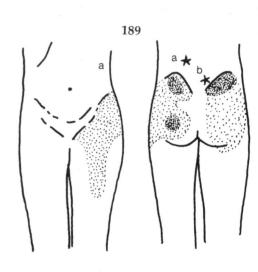

187 Dermatomes of the upper limb.

188 Dermatomes of the lower limb.

189 Pain patterns in (a) quadratus lumborum and (b) iliolumbar syndromes.

PAIN AND PAIN SYNDROMES

Innervation of apophyseal joints, outer annulus, longitudinal and short ligaments, and spinal dura is ultimately shared by the same spinal nerve, with considerable overlap between segments. Pain from spinal locomotor structures is thus poorly defined, with radiation over a wide area (which includes, potentially, the head, thorax, abdomen, and the upper or lower limb). The differential diagnosis of spinal syndromes may therefore be wide and embrace other systems.

'Mechanical' spinal pain

This heterogeneous group is by far the most common problem encountered. The pain is predominantly axial (unilateral, bilateral, or central) but may radiate into proximal or even distal limbs in an ill-defined, non-dermatomal pattern. It may be made worse by movement (usually in one plane) or prolonged standing or lifting, and is usually relieved by rest. On examination there may be painful restriction of movement in one direction more than another; a localised site of maximal tenderness (reproducing the pain); 'referred' tenderness and spasm of paraspinal muscles; and absence of neurological signs. In

many cases, anatomical localisation is difficult and no specific title can be given; in some cases, however, localised tenderness may permit labelling in anatomical terms (**189**).

Nerve root entrapment

Symptoms may be three-fold:

- Axial or unilateral proximal girdle pain from unilateral compression and tension of the dura mater.
- Root pain along part or all of the dermatome (variable between individuals) from pressure on dural sheath.
- Weakness, paraesthesiae and numbness due to nerve root (parenchymal) compression.

Root pain may occur on its own or be superimposed or follow mechanical back pain. It is characteristically sharp and shooting, and made worse by movement and increased intrathecal pressure (coughing, sneezing, straining at stool). Examination may reveal neurological signs (altered sensation, reduced power, reduced reflex) consistent with single root involvement.

Lumbar canal stenosis

This causes symptoms typical of low 'mechanical' back pain, except that:

- Paraesthesiae (non-dermatomal) occurs in one or both legs.
- Although symptoms worsen on activity, they may be absent or improve when the lumbar spine flexes forward, increasing the diameter of the canal (walking up steep inclines is better than down, cycling may cause no problems). The patient may adopt a 'simian' posture for this reason (hips, knees, lumbar spine slightly flexed).
- Neurological signs (decreased sensation, reflexes) may be present, though these may occur only after exercise.

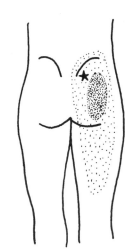

190 SIJ pain.

'Inflammatory' neck or back pain

This is characterised by diffuse axial pain and stiffness, worsened by rest, but improved by continuing exercise (initial movement may worsen it). Early morning and inactivity stiffness may be marked. Examination shows diffuse, symmetrical tenderness and muscle spasm, and restriction of movement in several or all directions. It may accompany sacroiliac symptoms or signs.

Sacroiliac pain

Characterised by diffuse, ill-defined pain in the ipsilateral buttock, radiating down the back of the leg (**190**), sacroiliac pain is worsened by stressing the joint, e.g. by running, or by standing on one leg.

'Bony pain'

Neck or back pain that is constant, severe, progressive, and present at night is very suggestive of malignancy or infection.

Referred pain

This may be from proximal locomotor structures (especially glenohumeral, hip joints), the major viscera, retroperitoneal structures, the urogenital system, or aorta. Associated features in the history and general examination should suggest the correct diagnosis; the pain shows no clear relationship to spinal movement; and examination of the spine is predominantly normal (referred *tenderness* can occur, but the patient's pain will not be reproduced by pressure on spinal structures).

EXAMINATION OF THE SPINE

The patient should be wearing only loose underwear. Inspect the standing patient from in front, from the side and from behind; inspect during walking: examine movements; then undertake palpation and appropriate neurological testing with the patient on a couch.

Inspection of the standing patient

Upper cervical and lumbar spinous processes normally lie deep within the spinal muscles: spinous processes of C7 ('vertebra prominens') and T1 (even more prominent) are most readily identified (**191**), and the thoracic spines are usually well seen, particularly on bending forward. After T1 the spine of each thoracic vertebra overlies the body of the vertebra below. The 'dimples of Venus' overlie the posterior iliac spines: a line between them overlies the S2 spinous process. The iliac crests may be visible (always palpable), and a line between these overlies the L4/5 interspace. The tip of the coccyx lies in the upper part of the natal cleft.

Look particularly for the following symptoms.

Loss of normal curves (cervical and lumbar lordosis, thoracic kyphosis)
Forward or lateral angulation of the head is common, resulting from diminished lower cervical lordosis and compensatory extension at the

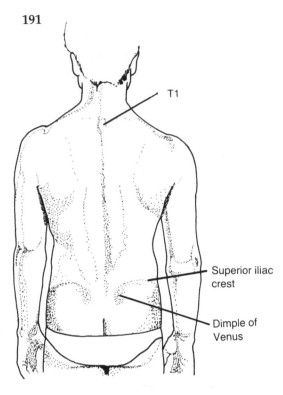

191 Normal surface landmarks (posterior view).

T1

Superior iliac crest

Dimple of Venus

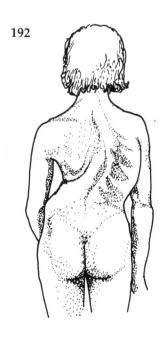

192 Scoliosis (right thoracic).

craniocervical junction: this may cause prominence of posterior muscles and horizontal skin folds below the occiput. Lateral angulation with rotation may accompany sternomastoid contracture, and several congenital abnormalities result in a short neck. If the thoracic spine shows excess forward angulation, note whether it is a smooth kyphosis (due to multisegment vertebral/disc disease) or sharply angulated (localised vertebral damage).

Scoliosis
Its site is represented by the apex of the curve (thoracic, thoracolumbar, or lumbar), its laterality by the side of the convexity (**192**). Scoliosis may be *compensated* (T1 centred over sacrum) or *uncompensated* (a perpendicular from T1 lying outside the sacrum). *Postural scoliosis* (no intrinsic bony abnormality in spine or ribs) resolves as the patient flexes forwards; by contrast, *structural scoliosis* persists or is accentuated by flexion. With thoracic scoliosis, rotation of vertebrae may produce a hump or 'gibbus' of the ribs on the convex side. *Pelvic tilt* (iliac crests at different heights ± asymmetry of gluteal folds) may accompany scoliosis or relate to leg shortening, or to hip or other lower limb arthropathy. 'Sciatic' scoliosis resulting from spinal pain is postural and usually mild.

Reduced chest movement
Usually resulting from intrathoracic disease, reduced chest movement may also occur with arthropathy. If expansion appears reduced, measure from full expiration to full inspiration at the nipple line, with the patient's arms on or behind their head (normally 4 cm or more in the adult male).

Paraspinal muscle spasm
The muscles look as though they are bulging out alongside the spinous processes. Spasm may be unilateral or bilateral, and may associate with spasm of ipsilateral buttock muscles (especially with sciatic pain due to disc prolapse).

Skin changes
Moles, vascular malformations, and hairy tufts may indicate the site of underlying congenital abnormalities of vertebral bodies. Note any scars or nodules (most common over the bony prominences).

Inspection of the walking patient

With low-back problems the pelvis may not rotate fully with the advancing leg, remaining mainly aligned with the thorax. This gives a shortened step, jerkiness of movement, and considerable caution and awkwardness when turning. SIJ pain may be worsened by weight bearing and is particularly provoked by standing on one (the ipsilateral) leg.

Inspection during movement

As far as possible it is best to isolate movements at different segments. Look for any asymmetry, restriction, or pain on movement.

Lumbar movements

With the patient still standing, the examiner places the fingers of one hand over consecutive lumbar spinous processes and asks the patient to bend forward to touch the toes (this also involves hip flexion). The lumbar lordosis should be replaced by a smooth curve, the degree of movement indicated by separation of the examiner's fingers (193). If present, observe any change in scoliosis. Then, stabilising the pelvis firmly with both hands, ask the patient to bend backwards (extension; 194), and then slide their hand down each leg (lateral flexion — lumbar and thoracic segments; 195).

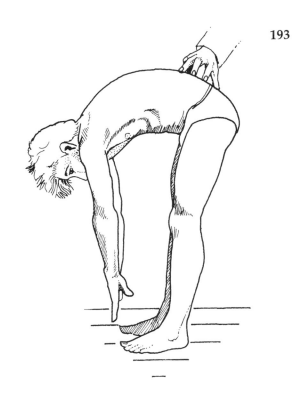

193 Thoracolumbar flexion.

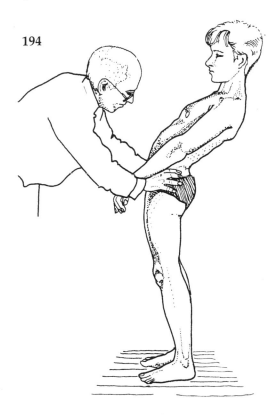

194 Extension.

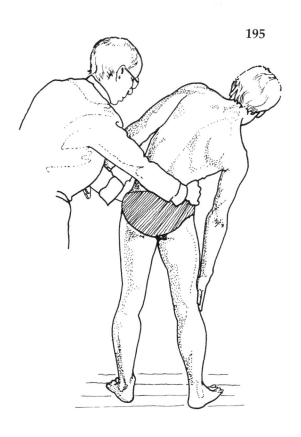

195 Lateral flexion.

Thoracolumbar rotation and cervical movements

For these, fix the shoulder girdles to the trunk by getting the patient to clasp their arms across their chest, and fix the pelvis by firmly holding each iliac crest (with the patient's feet apart) or, preferably, by seating the patient astride a chair. Ask the patient to turn round as far as possible to each

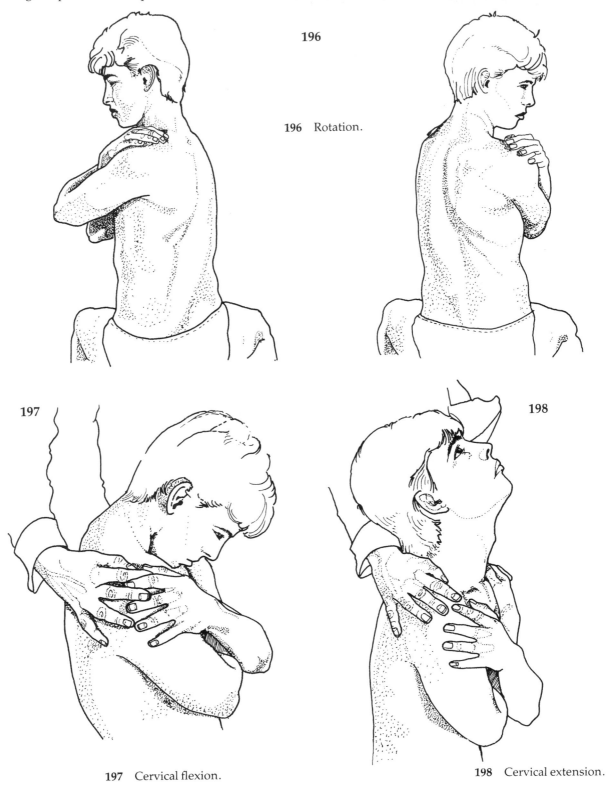

196

196 Rotation.

197 Cervical flexion.

198 Cervical extension.

side (rotation — mainly thoracic, **196**). Then, holding the patient's 'fixed' shoulders, ask the patient to put their chin on their chest (flexion, **197**), look up in the air (extension, **198**), look round to each side (rotation, **199**), and then put each ear over onto the shoulder (lateral flexion, **200**). During lateral flexion, pain felt on the side to which the head moves suggests facet joint disease, whereas pain on the opposite side is more likely muscle spasm.

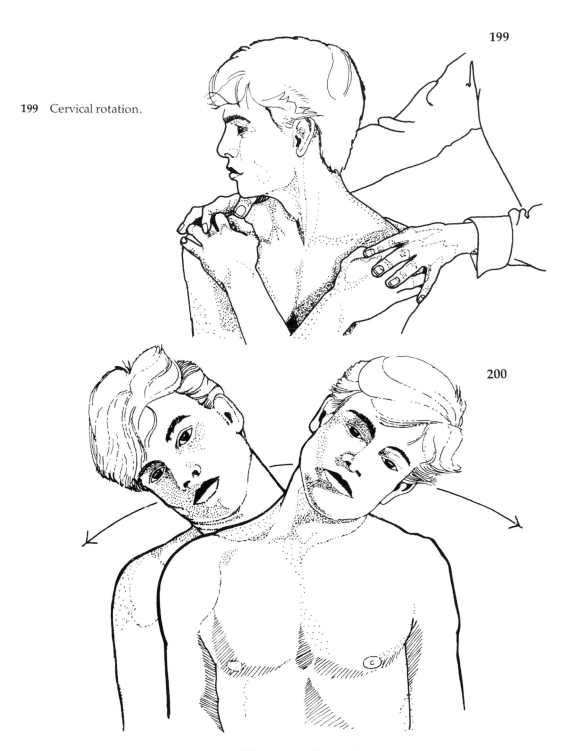

199   Cervical rotation.

199

200

200   Cervical lateral flexion.

Palpation

Lay the patient face down on the couch, relaxed with arms folded underneath. For palpation of the neck, place a pillow under the upper chest; for the thoracic and lumbar spine, move the pillow under the abdomen — this helps to relax the muscles, supports the spine in flexion, and aids separation of the spinous processes (**201, 202**). Palpate in turn the following areas:

- *Skin and subcutaneous tissues.* Palpate in a line down each side of the trunk. Use a 'skin rolling' technique (**203**), to look for areas of hyperaesthesiae. This is a useful but poor localising sign suggesting possible pathology in the nearby region of the spine (analogous to generalised abdominal tenderness with appendicitis).
- *The paraspinal muscles.* Feel for increased tone and tenderness on one or both sides (**204**). This again is a poor localising sign.

- *The interspinous ligaments.* Apply firm pressure over each in turn (**205**). Tenderness with reproduction of the patient's pain suggests local ligamentous or disc disease. Other abnormalities to note during palpation include defects in the spinous processes (spina bifida occulta), or a 'step' deformity of spondylolisthesis (usually L4/5) or retrolisthesis (more common in the cervical spine).
- *The facet joints.* Applying firm, jarring pressure with each thumb just lateral to the spinous process (**206**) may cause pain relating to local facet joint, disc, or ligament lesions.
- *Mid-trapezius.* This is palpated for hyperalgesia of fibromyalgia syndrome.
- *The medial iliac crest.* This is a common site of tenderness, with reproduction of the patient's pain ('iliolumbar' or 'iliac crest syndrome').

201

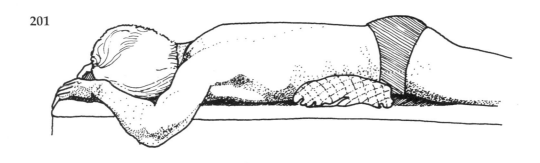

202

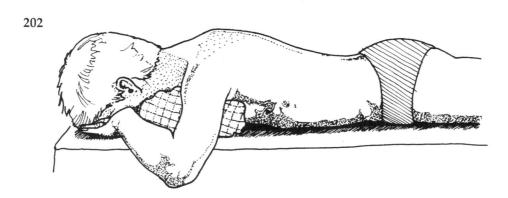

201, 202   Position for palpation of (**201**) back and (**202**) neck.

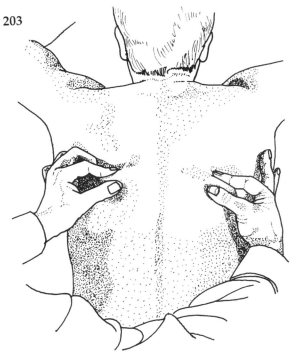

203 'Skin rolling' for hyperaesthesia.

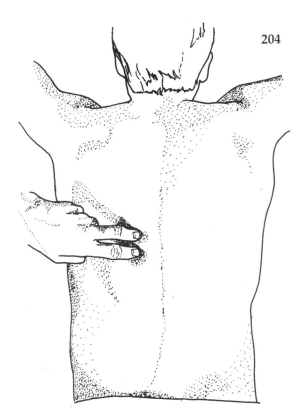

204 Palpation of paraspinal muscles.

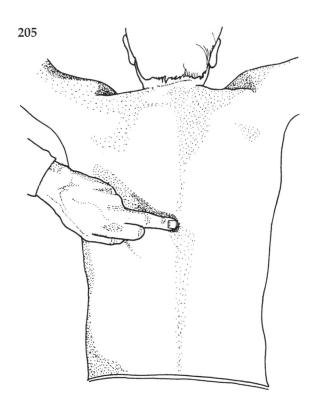

205 Palpation of interspinous processes.

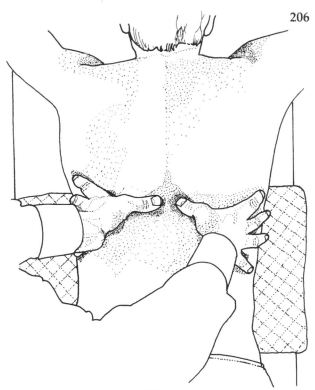

206 Palpation for facet joint tenderness.

Examination of the SIJ

The SIJ, which is inaccessible to palpation, is difficult to assess clinically. Only florid inflammation or damage to the fibrous portion is likely to result in local tenderness posteriorly (most such tenderness is probably ligamentous). Tests designed to stress the SIJs and reproduce pain in the buttock are non-specific and include:

- *Distraction tests.* Firm downward pressure over both sides of the pelvis with the patient lying supine (**207**), or over the pelvis with the patient lying on one side (**208**).
- *'Knee-to-shoulder' test* (**209**). With the patient lying flat, flex and adduct one hip and push the flexed knee towards the opposite shoulder, stressing the ipsilateral SIJ. This test is helpful only if the hip and lumbar spine are normal.

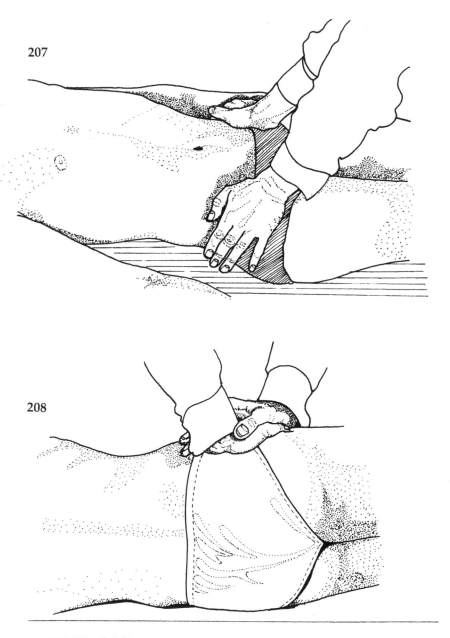

207

208

207, 208   SIJ distraction tests: (**207**) patient supine; (**208**) patient on side.

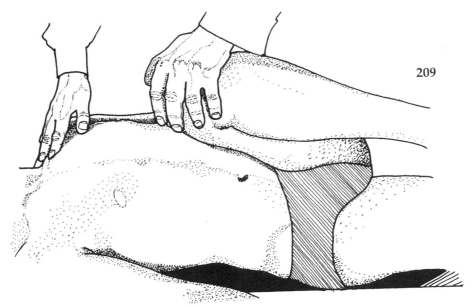

209 Knee-to-shoulder test.

Neurological aspects

Provocation tests for root lesions

Numerous named tests exist, all using man-oeuvres to distract roots or increase intrathecal pressure and thus reproduce the patient's symptoms.

Straight leg raising (SLR, Lasègue's test)

The most common test used. With the patient lying flat on the back and completely relaxed, slowly raise the straightened leg on the affected side by 70°, maintaining full extension at the knee, until the patient complains of pain or tightness down the leg (**210–212**). Note the angle of elevation, then drop the leg back slightly to eliminate the pain. Now ask the patient to flex the neck by putting the chin on the chest, or passively dorsiflex the raised foot. Reproduction of pain by either action indicates stretching of the dura (a central prolapse often causing back > leg pain, a lateral prolapse the reverse); SLR pain not reproduced by these actions suggests hamstring pain (mainly posterior thigh) or lumbar or sacro-iliac pain (felt more in the back than the leg).

During elevation of the leg from 0 to 40°, there is no traction on the roots but 'slack' in the sciatic arborisation is taken up; between 40 and 70°, there is tension applied to the roots (mainly L5, S1, and S2); above 70°, no further root deformation occurs, and any pain after this elevation is probably articular. Compare both legs for any difference. Reproduction of pain in the affected side by elevation of the opposite leg ('cross-over sign' or

'well leg raise test') indicates thecal compression by an often large lesion medial to the nerve root (disc or tumour). If both legs are raised together ('*bilateral SLR*'), little distortion of nerve roots occurs; pain appearing before 70° probably arises from SIJs, pain beyond 70° from the lumbar spine (**213**).

Femoral nerve stretch test

This produces traction on the L2, L3, and L4 nerve roots. Lay the patient on the unaffected side with the affected hip and knee slightly flexed, the back straight and the head flexed. Gently extend the hip and increase knee flexion; pain down the anterior thigh indicates a positive test (**214**). As with SLR, a contralateral positive test may also occur.

Neurological examination for root abnormality

The principal abnormalities of sensation, power, and reflexes accompanying individual root lesions are summarised in *Tables 9* and *10*.

Examination for cord signs

A spastic gait, lower limb ataxia, increased reflexes, and extensor plantar responses (i.e. upper motor neurone signs) indicate pressure or damage to the cord, the level being determined principally by the division between normal and abnormal reflexes and the level of any accompanying lower neurone signs.

210–212 SLR test: (**210**) elevate to cause pain; (**211**) lower the leg, then dorsiflex the foot; or (**212**) flex the head.

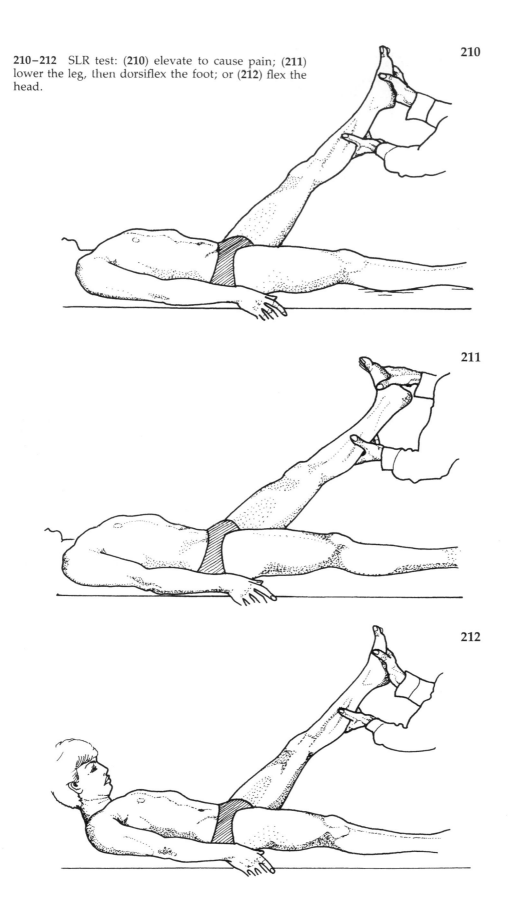

210

211

212

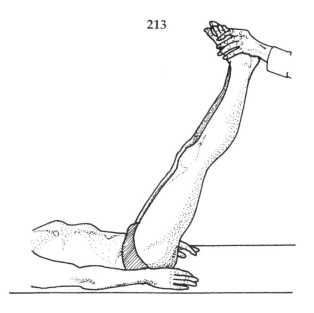

213

213 Bilateral SLR.

Table 9. Principal cervical root syndromes (affected dermatomes, myotomes, and reflexes).

Root	Sensation	Weakness	Reflex
C5	Lateral upper arm	Shoulder abduction	Biceps
C6	Lateral forearm	Elbow flexion, wrist extension	Brachio-radialis
C7	Middle finger	Elbow extension, wrist flexion	Triceps
C8	Medial forearm	Thumb extension, ulnar deviation of wrist	—
T1	Medial elbow region	Hand intrinsics, finger ab/adduction	—

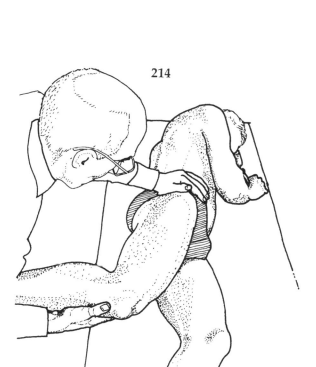

214

214 Femoral nerve stretch test.

Table 10. Principal lumbar root syndromes (affected dermatomes, myotomes, and reflexes).

Root	Sensation	Weakness	Reflex
L4	Anterior leg, medial foot	Ankle dorsiflexion (tibialis anterior)	Knee jerk
L5	Lateral leg/thigh, web of hallux	Extension of great toe (ext. hallucis longus)	—
S1	Posterior leg, lateral foot	Eversion of foot (peroneals)	Ankle jerk

Assessment of power, plantar responses, and sensation may be difficult in patients with polyarthritis and joint deformity, muscle wasting, and entrapment or peripheral neuropathy. Upper cervical cord damage due to C1/2 instability in rheumatoid arthritis is a particular problem: helpful signs in this situation may include positive pectoralis jerks (**215**; suggesting a lesion above C4), a normal jaw jerk (implying a lesion below the brainstem), and diminished/absent corneal reflex (the sensory part of the fifth cranial nerve centre extends into the upper cervical cord).

Examination of other systems

Pain in the spine may be referred, and a thorough assessment of other systems (particularly the lower bowel and genital tract) may be required in individual cases.

Additional tests/procedures

Measurements of spinal movements

In addition to simply assessing distraction of fingers placed on spinous processes, thoracolumbar flexion can be estimated by the *modified Schober test* (216). Get the patient as flexed as possible (standing or sitting) and, starting from an upper sacral spinous prominence, mark out three 10cm segments up the spine. Then remeasure the distances between the marks with the patient erect: the lowest segment should shorten by at least 50%, the middle by 40%, the upper by 30% (shortening is greater in tall subjects). An alternative is to measure the C7–T12 and T12–S1 distances erect and then during maximal flexion; the thoracic measurement should increase 2–3cm, the lumbar distance 7–8 cm.

Other measurements employed include the *finger-to-floor* distance when the standing patient attempts to touch the floor with legs straight; and the *occiput-to-wall distance*, measured with the patient standing upright, heels back against a wall, eyes level.

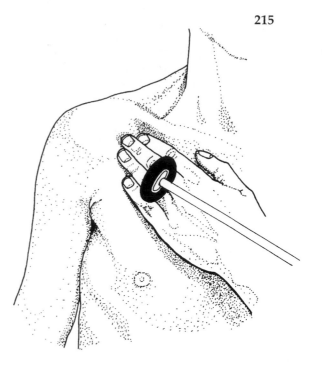

215

215   Pectoralis jerk.

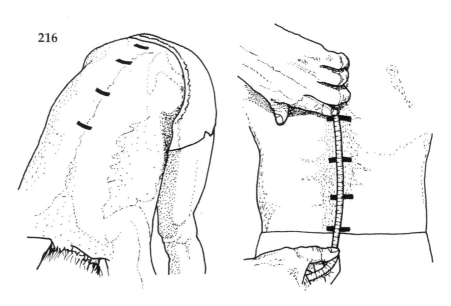

216

216   Modified Schober test.

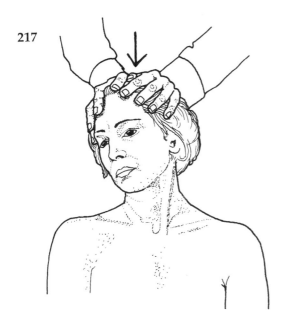

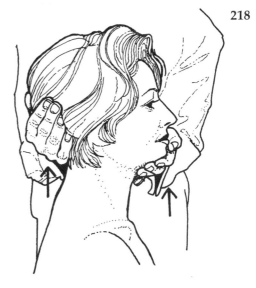

218 Cervical distraction.

217 Foraminal compression test.

Foraminal compression/distraction tests

These may be used for cervical entrapment syndromes, but are rarely positive. Passively rotate and laterally flex the neck towards the affected side, then carefully press down on the head; reproduction of pain down the arm or around the scapula region suggests root entrapment or facet joint disease (*foraminal compression test*; **217**). Conversely, upward traction on the neck, by lifting with one hand under the chin and the other under the occiput, may relieve pain due to root compression (*distraction test*; **218**).

Milgram's and Hoover's tests

These are used to distinguish 'organic' from 'functional' pain. In *Milgram's test* the supine patient performs active bilateral SLR to a height of 6 inches. This greatly increases thecal pressure and ability to hold this position for any time excludes significant thecal pathology. In *Hoover's test* the patient performs unilateral SLR with the examiner's hand under the other heel; absence of downward heel pressure indicates that the patient is not really trying (**219**).

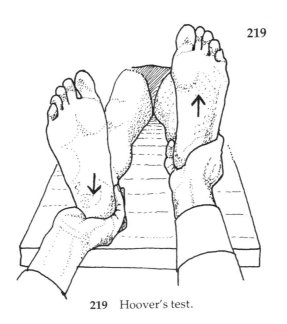

219 Hoover's test.

SUMMARY OF EXAMINATION OF SPINE

(1) Inspection of the standing patient
    (a) from in front (head angulation, chest expansion)
    (b) from the side (spinal curves)
    (c) from behind (scoliosis, pelvic tilt, muscles, skin)
(2) Inspection of the walking patient
(3) Inspection during movement (restriction, pain)
    (a) standing
        flexion – 'touch toes' (± modified Schober test)
        extension
        lateral flexion
    (b) preferably sitting astride chair
        thoracolumbar rotation
        cervical flexion, extension, lateral flexion, rotation
(4) Palpation of patient lying on couch
    (a) 'skin rolling' each side (hyperaesthesia)
    (b) paraspinal muscles (tone, tenderness)
    (c) interspinous ligaments (pain)
    (d) facet joint region (pain)
    (e) medial iliac crest (tenderness)
(5) Stressing of sacroiliac joints
    (a) distraction
    (b) knee-to-shoulder test
(6) Provocation tests for root entrapment
    (a) straight leg raising each side
    (b) bilateral SLR
    (c) femoral nerve stretch test
(7) Neurological examination (power, reflexes, sensation)
(8) Detailed examination of other systems as required

7   Hip

The hip is a large ball-and-socket joint that plays a major role in weight bearing, stance and locomotion (walking, running, jumping, swimming, etc.). It thus needs to permit a *wide range of movement* while maintaining *great stability*. Mobility is aided by the elongated femoral neck which offsets the shaft from the head, an arrangement which also gives great leverage to muscles acting at the proximal femur. Stability is due to:

- The powerful muscles acting across the hip.
- The strong fibrous capsule.
- The deep insertion of the femoral head into the acetabulum.

Forces across each hip are often great: for example, standing on both feet (one-third body weight), standing on one leg (2.5 × body weight), or walking (1.5–6 × body weight). Under low loads the joint surfaces are incongruous, but under heavy loads they become congruous, providing maximum surface contact to keep the load/unit area within tolerable limits.

The *acetabular cavity* is formed at the meeting point of the three bones comprising the innominate (the ileum, the ischium, and the pubis: **220, 221**).

It opens outwards, forwards, and downwards, and is strongest superiorly and posteriorly (where it is subject to greatest strain in the erect or stooped position). The rim is deepened by the fibrocartilaginous labrum, which forms a collar around the femoral head, narrowing the outlet and stabilising the head within the acetabulum. A gap in the lower portion of the labrum, the acetabular notch, is bridged by the transverse ligament, converting the notch into a foramen through which blood vessels pass into the joint. The articular cartilage is horseshoe shaped with the open part pointing inferiorly; a fat mass fills the fossa at the bottom of the acetabulum. Hyaline cartilage covers the whole of the femoral head except at the attachment of ligamentum teres, where there is a small bony defect, the fovea.

The strong, dense fibrous *capsule* arises circumferentially from the acetabulum, labrum, and transverse ligament. It attaches distally to the intertrochanteric line of the femur anteriorly, and about half-way along the neck posteriorly. It is reinforced in front by the Y-shaped iliofemoral ligament (the strongest in the body), inferiorly by the pubofemoral ligament, and posteriorly by the

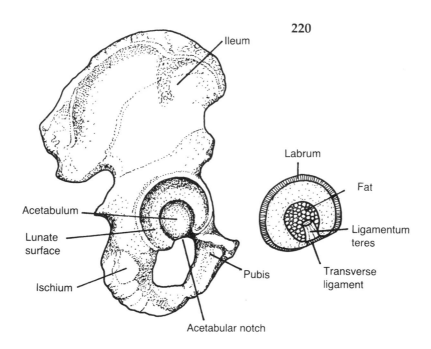

220   Bony contours of the acetabulum. The inset shows the arrangement of the labrum, transverse ligament, ligamentum, and central fat.

221 Section through the hip joint.

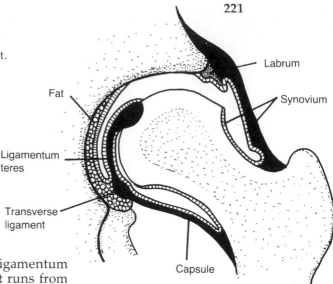

ischiofemoral ligament (**222**). The ligamentum teres is an intracapsular ligament that runs from the transverse ligament to the fovea: it has no joint stabilising function but carries blood vessels which supply a small area of the head around the fovea. The synovium lines the capsule, labrum and fat pad, and excludes the ligamentum teres; distally, it reflects onto the femoral neck and extends to the cartilage of the head. The iliotibial band is part of the fascia lata, extending from its main attachment at the iliac crest to the lateral tibial tubercle. Clinically relevant *bursae* (**223**) around the hip include:

- The large, often multilocular, trochanteric bursa between the greater trochanter and gluteus maximus.
- The iliopectineal bursa between the anterior capsule and iliopsoas (communicating with the joint in about 15%).
- The ischiogluteal bursa over the ischial tuberosity, overlying the sciatic nerve.

The strong muscles around the hip have complex actions, and hip movements are influenced by the position of the lumbar spine, the knee, and the opposite hip (e.g. flexion increases if the knee and spine also flex; extension increases if the knee is extended; abduction increases if both hips are slightly flexed). The prime movers are:

Flexors:	iliopsoas (L2, 3 nerve root supply)	
	(pectineus, rectus femoris)	
Extensors:	gluteus maximus,	(L4, 5; S1, 2)
	hamstrings	
Abductors:	gluteus medius	(L4, 5; S1)
	(gluteus minimus)	
Adductors:	adductor longus,	(L3, 4, 5; S1)
	magnus, brevis	
Rotation		
External:	piriformis, obturator,	(L4, 5; S1)
	gemelli, gluteus medius	
Internal:	gluteus minimus,	(L4, 5; S1)
	gluteus medius, tensor fascia latae	

222

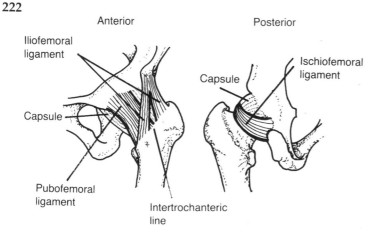

222 Joint capsule and ligaments.

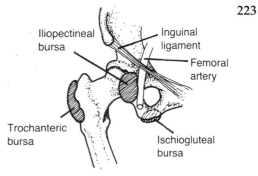

223

223 Clinically important bursae.

Important structures adjacent to the joint include the neurovascular bundle anteriorly, and the sciatic nerve running close to the posterior aspect.

In the adult the hip is an important site of involvement in osteoarthritis and, less commonly, other major arthropathies: periarticular lesions (bursitis, enthesopathy) are common. In the neonate and child, congenital dislocation, Perthes' disease, slipped femoral epiphysis, and sepsis are the principal conditions.

SYMPTOMS

The hip joint is formed largely from the L3 segment. Hip pain is often ill-defined, worsened by loading and movement (e.g. rising from sitting, standing, walking, putting on socks), and felt primarily in the anterior groin (**224**). However, it may radiate widely to the anterior and lateral aspects of the thigh, the buttock, the anterior aspect of the knee, and rarely down the front of the shin to above the ankle. Presentation may be with isolated knee pain (the hip and knee both contribute fibres to the obturator and femoral nerves).

Because of its wide and variable radiation, hip pain requires differentiation from a number of other local or distant causes, including:

- *Sacroiliac pain.* This is felt deep in the buttock, with variable radiation down the posterior thigh. It is often exacerbated by standing on one leg (the affected side: p. 81).
- *Bursitis.* Trochanteric bursitis causes localised pain and tenderness over the trochanter, with occasional radiation down the lateral thigh. It is particularly painful when lying on the affected side (e.g. in bed). Pain from ischiogluteal bursitis is felt mainly posteriorly and is particularly worsened by sitting.

- *Enthesopathy.* Adductor enthesopathy ('groin strain') usually follows a sporting injury and causes pain in the medial groin, worsened by standing on the affected leg. Abductor enthesopathy produces similar pain to trochanteric bursitis, but is usually worsened by walking.
- *Meralgia paraesthetica.* Entrapment neuropathy of the lateral cutaneous nerve of the thigh (beneath the inguinal ligament) causes burning pain and numbness over the anterolateral thigh. It may accompany massive or rapid-onset obesity, pregnancy, and wearing of tight corsets or jeans.
- *Root pain.* Prolapsed intervertebral discs or lesions involving L1/L2 nerve roots (both rare) may produce groin pain (**225**). Its sharp quality and exacerbation by straining/coughing (± accompanying back pain) help suggest its nature.
- *Symphysitis.* This may produce supra-pubic pain and tenderness, worse during the stance phase of walking.

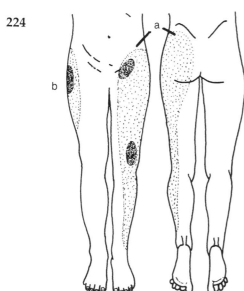

224 Pain distribution in (a) hip disease and (b) trochanteric bursitis.

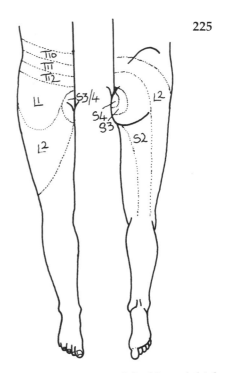

225 Dermatomes around the hip and thigh.

EXAMINATION

The patient, undressed to underwear, is examined standing, walking, and then lying.

Inspection of the standing patient

Ask the patient to point to the site of maximum pain and to delineate the area over which pain is felt. Inspect from in front, the side, and from behind.

Readily identifiable landmarks include the *iliac crests*, running between the *anterior* and *posterior superior iliac spines*, the *greater trochanters*, the *ischial tuberosities*, the *gluteal folds*, and the

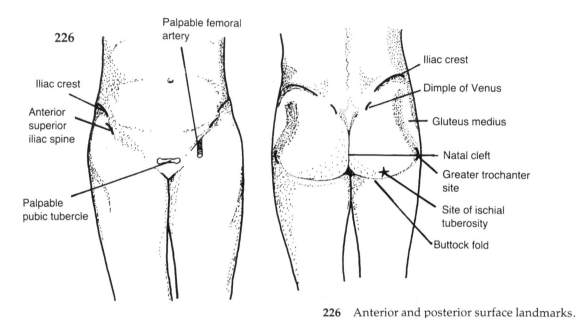

226 Anterior and posterior surface landmarks.

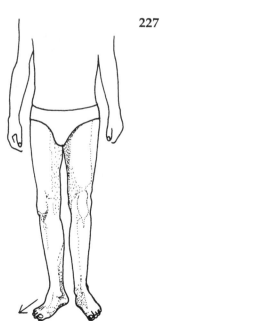

227 Rotational deformity.

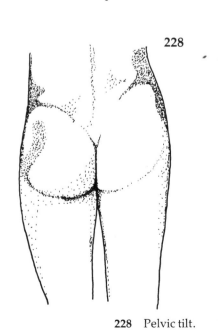

228 Pelvic tilt.

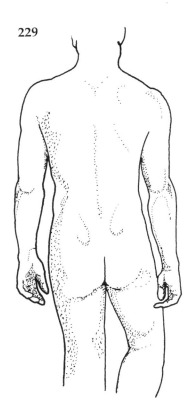
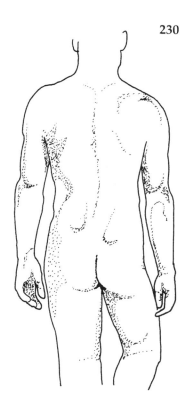

229,230 The Trendelenburg test: (**229**) normal; (**230**) abnormal.

rounded proximal buttock muscles (**226**). From in front, look particularly for:

- *Pelvic tilt* — shown by loss of level between the anterior superior iliac spines. This may be due to adduction or abduction deformity from hip disease, a short leg, or primary scoliosis.
- *Rotational deformity* (**227**) — see whether the feet face forwards to the same degree.

From the side, look particularly for:

- *Exaggerated lumbar lordosis* — this may indicate a fixed flexion deformity of one or both hips.

From behind, look particularly for:

- *Pelvic tilt* (**228**) — shown by loss of level between the iliac crests, and asymmetry of the gluteal folds. With fixed adduction, the abnormal side is elevated and the patient may be unable to place the ipsilateral foot flat on the floor. With an abduction deformity, the situation is reversed.

- *Scoliosis* — this often accompanies pelvic tilt.
- *Muscle wasting* — secondary to hip, primary muscle or neurological disease.

The *Trendelenburg test* shows up gross weakness of the hip abductors (gluteus medius, minimus). Ask the patient to lift one foot off the ground (**229, 230**). Normally, to retain balance, the abductors on the weight-bearing side contract to elevate the unsupported side. If the abductors are weak, the pelvis may drop down on the contralateral side: the patient may lose balance, stumble, and be unable to keep the foot raised. A modification is to stand facing the patient, providing support by holding the hands; as the foot is raised it is easy to appreciate the increased load transmitted from the patient with weak abductors. The common causes of a positive Trendelenburg test are hip disease (unilateral or bilateral), an L5 root lesion (unilateral), and conditions characterised by generalised weakness (usually bilateral).

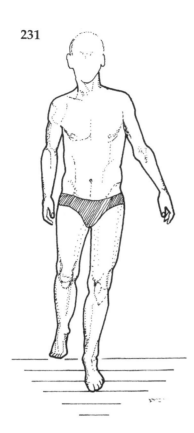

231

Inspection of the walking patient

Two non-specific gait abnormalities commonly result from hip disease:

- *Antalgic gait* (p. 24; **231**) — usually indicating a painful hip. The patient shortens stance phase on the affected hip, leaning over the affected side to avoid painful contraction of the hip abductors.
- *Trendelenburg gait* ('abductor limp'; **232**) — indicating weakness of the abductors on the affected side. During the stance phase on the affected side, the contralateral pelvis dips down and the body leans to the unaffected side. If bilateral, this produces a 'waddling gait'.

231 Antalgic gait.

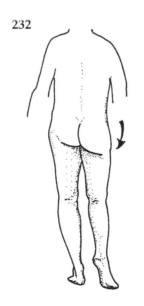

232

232 Trendelenburg gait.

Inspection of the patient lying on a couch

The patient, in general, should be lying straight out, as flat as is compatible with cardiorespiratory function. Ensure that both anterior superior iliac spines are level and the two legs are aligned.

Inspection

Look particularly for:

- *Skin changes* (especially scars, inguinal rash).
- *Swelling.* Swelling of the iliopectineal bursa may occasionally be apparent in the medial aspect of the groin. The hip joint is deep and swelling is usually not apparent. Anteromedial swelling extending down the thigh may occur with large synovial (Baker's) cyst extensions.
- *Deformity* — particularly fixed flexion, external rotation or abduction deformity (these often accumulate sequentially as hip disease progresses; **233**). With a severe flexion deformity the patient will be unable to straighten the legs without sitting up. With fixed adduction the affected leg may cross the other. Rotational deformities are obvious by looking at the position of the patella and feet on the two sides.

  Restricted hip flexion may be compensated by an increase in lumbar lordosis which then 'masks' the fixed flexion deformity. If fixed flexion is not readily apparent utilise *Thomas' test* (**234**). Flex the other hip to 90° to eliminate the lumbar lordosis (confirmed by placing a hand under the patient's lumbar spine) and watch for flexion of the affected hip.

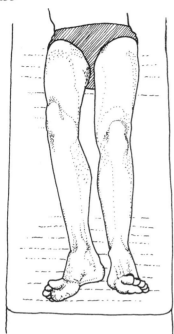

233 Deformities: fixed flexion, external rotation, abduction.

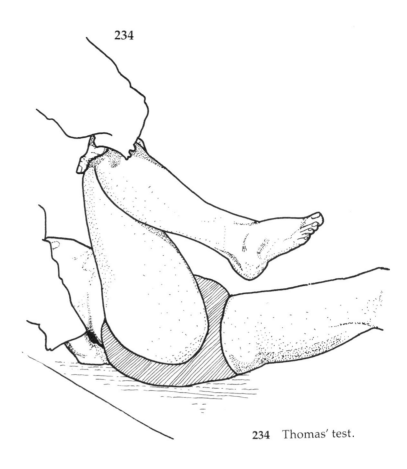

234 Thomas' test.

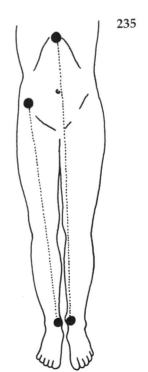

235 True and apparent leg length.

- *Leg length inequality* — apparent by looking at the heels. If there is apparent discrepancy use a soft tape measure to estimate on each side:

  (a) the *true leg length* — between the anterior superior iliac spine and the medial malleolus (**235**). If one leg is flexed or externally rotated the other must be positioned similarly before measurement. Shortening (>1 cm) is often due to, but is not specific to, hip disease.

  (b) the *apparent leg length* — from the medial malleolus to a fixed point on the trunk (the xiphisternum is more 'fixed' than the umbilicus; in children the manubriosternal junction is more readily palpable). Inequality most commonly results from pelvic tilt.

- *Attitude* — a painful hip with synovitis is most comfortable if held in mild flexion, abduction, and external rotation. Observe if this is the position the patient keeps wanting to adopt.

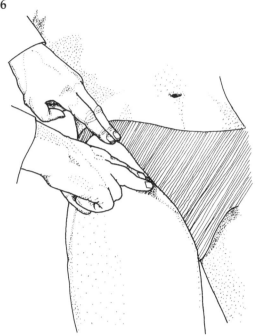

236

236 Palpation of anterior joint-line region.

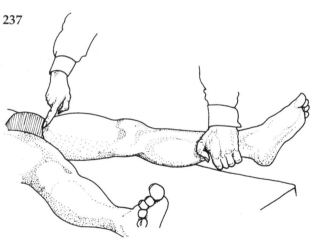

237

237 Resisted active adduction and site of tenderness in adductor enthesopathy.

238 Palpation of trochanteric bursitis and abductor enthesopathy.

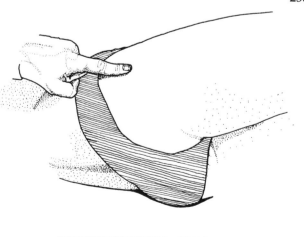

238

Palpation

Palpate for tenderness (± swelling) over the following areas:

- With the patient supine, palpate the *anterior joint line* just lateral to the femoral artery pulsation, below the middle third of the inguinal ligament (**236**). Tenderness here may reflect hip *synovitis* or *iliopectineal bursitis*. Bursal swelling may be palpable and give a positive balloon sign (reflecting localised bursitis or a synovial cyst communicating with an inflamed joint). Bursal swelling requires differentiation from other swellings in this region (particularly femoral hernia — usually medial to the artery). Tenderness over the *adductor origins* along the superior or inferior aspect of the pubic bone may reflect adductor enthesopathy: resisted active adduction (**237**) may reproduce the pain.
- With the patient on their side palpate around the greater trochanter for tenderness due to *trochanteric bursitis* or *abductor enthesopathy* (**238**). In obese subjects locate the trochanter by feeling proximally up the femur. Active abduction of the affected leg (alone or against resistance) may reproduce the pain of abductor enthesopathy (**239**), but will not usually worsen bursitis.
- With the patient still on their side, flex their knee and hip and feel for the prominent ischial tuberosity (**240**). Tenderness here suggests *ischiogluteal bursitis* (this is also an infrequent site for rheumatoid nodules).

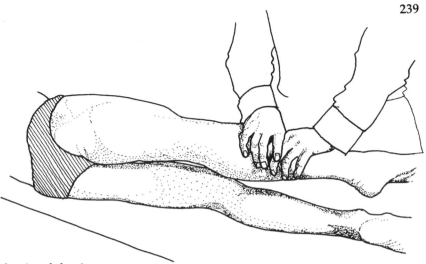

239 Resisted active abduction.

Movements

With the exception of extension, hip movements are best tested with the patient supine. Look for restriction and presence of pain for each movement in turn.

- *Flexion* (about 120°). This is tested with the knee flexed to relax the hamstrings (**241**).

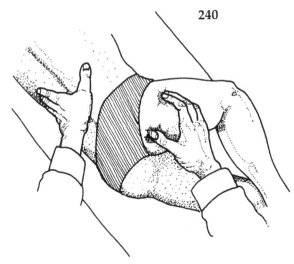

240 Palpation of ischial tuberosity and ischiogluteal bursitis.

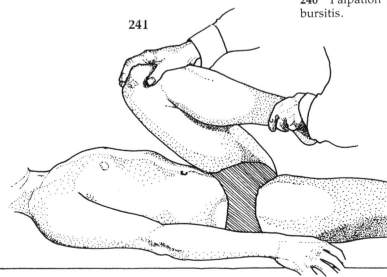

241 Hip flexion.

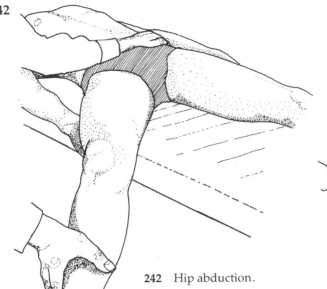

242 Hip abduction.

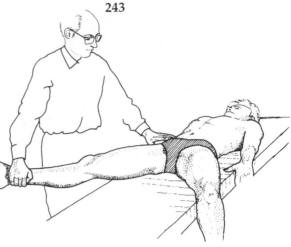

243 Hip abduction with pelvis fixed.

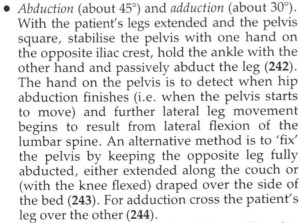

244 Hip adduction.

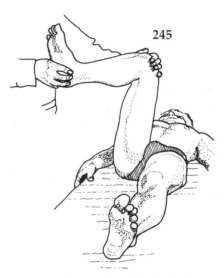

245 Internal rotation in flexion.

- *Abduction* (about 45°) and *adduction* (about 30°). With the patient's legs extended and the pelvis square, stabilise the pelvis with one hand on the opposite iliac crest, hold the ankle with the other hand and passively abduct the leg (**242**). The hand on the pelvis is to detect when hip abduction finishes (i.e. when the pelvis starts to move) and further lateral leg movement begins to result from lateral flexion of the lumbar spine. An alternative method is to 'fix' the pelvis by keeping the opposite leg fully abducted, either extended along the couch or (with the knee flexed) draped over the side of the bed (**243**). For adduction cross the patient's leg over the other (**244**).
- *Internal* and *external rotation* (about 45° each). Flex the hip and knee to 90° and move the foot out laterally (internal rotation; **245**) and medially (external rotation; **246**). Internal rotation in

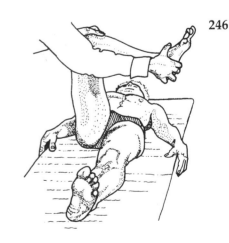

246 External rotation in flexion.

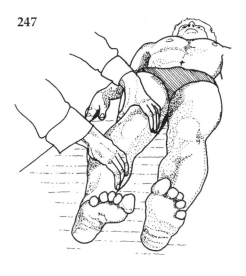

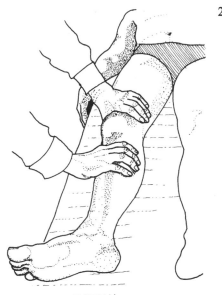

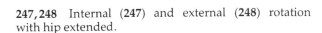

247,248 Internal (**247**) and external (**248**) rotation with hip extended.

flexion is the earliest and most constant movement to be affected by hip disease. Rotation can also be assessed with the hip extended and the leg straight: roll each leg on the couch, first one way and then the other, looking at the foot as an indicator of rotation (**247, 248**).

- *Extension* (about 15°). Thomas' test detects loss of extension (i.e. fixed flexion). For smaller losses of extension lay the patient prone and attempt to immobilise the pelvis by downward pressure with one hand (over the sacrum) while extending the hip with the other hand (under the thigh: **249**). If the patient has difficulty lying prone, lay them on their side and get them to flex the lower leg and hold it firmly (to stabilise the pelvis); stand behind the patient and support the upper leg while extending the hip, checking with the other hand over the lumbosacral junction for any spinal/pelvic movement.

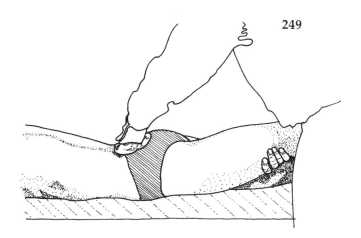

249 Extension assessed in prone position.

SUMMARY OF HIP EXAMINATION

(1) Inspection of the standing patient
    (a) from in front (pelvic tilt, rotational deformity)
    (b) from the side (increased lumbar lordosis)
    (c) from behind (pelvic tilt, scoliosis, wasting)
        Trendelenburg test
(2) Inspection of the walking patient (antalgic, Trendelenburg gait)
(3) Inspection of the patient lying on a couch
    (a) inspection:
        skin
        swelling
        deformity
        Thomas' test (fixed flexion)
        leg length inequality (true + apparent leg length)
    (b) palpation:
        anterior joint line
        adductor origins
        greater trochanter (patient on side)
        ischial tuberosity (patient on side)
    (c) movements:
        flexion
        abduction, adduction
        internal, external rotation
        extension (patient prone or on side)

8 Knee

The knee is the largest synovial joint and contains the largest sesamoid (the patella). The three compartments (medial and lateral tibiofemoral and patellofemoral) share a common cavity (250). The suprapatellar synovial reflection (pouch) is more extensive on the medial aspect and offers little resistance to fluid distension. Posteriorly, in the popliteal fossa, the synovial cavity is more constrained; its contour is moulded by tendons into convoluted recesses, the largest of which are the semimembranosus and lateral and medial gastrocnemius bursae and the subpopliteal recess (all of which communicate with the main cavity). Non-communicating bursae also occur, the most important clinically being the prepatellar bursa, the superficial and deep infrapatellar bursae (251), and the anserine bursa (252).

The two fibrocartilage menisci (semilunar cartilages) are important load-transmitting structures (253). The medial meniscus has a thickened outer

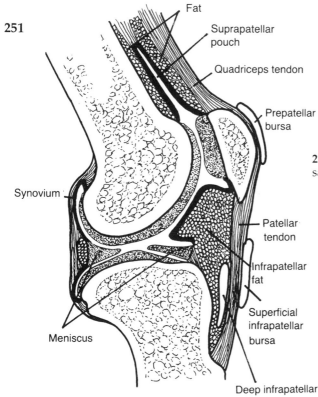

250 Knee compartments.

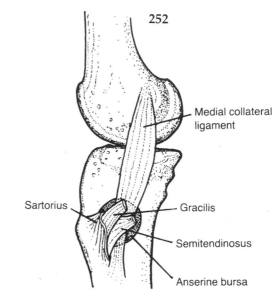

252 Medial collateral ligament and sites of insertion of sartorius, gracilis, and semitendinosus.

251 Synovial contour and non-communicating bursae.

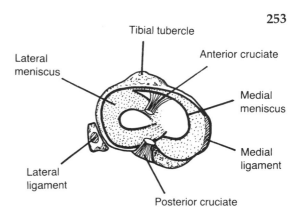

253 Medial and lateral menisci.

107

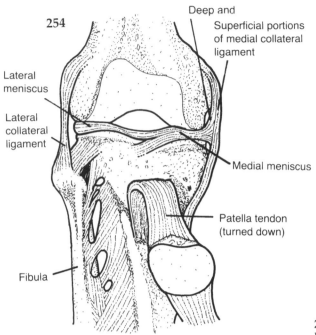

254

Deep and Superficial portions of medial collateral ligament

Lateral meniscus

Lateral collateral ligament

Medial meniscus

Patella tendon (turned down)

Fibula

254   Collateral ligaments viewed from in front.

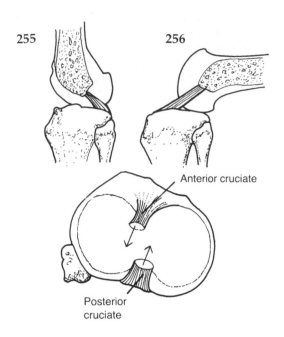

255   **256**

Anterior cruciate

Posterior cruciate

255,256   Posterior (**255**) and anterior (**256**) cruciate ligaments viewed from the side and from above.

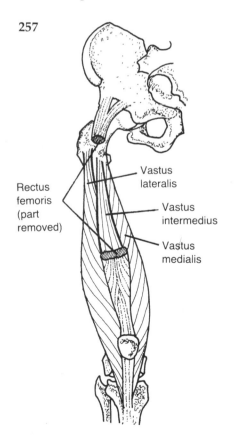

257

Rectus femoris (part removed)

Vastus lateralis

Vastus intermedius

Vastus medialis

257   The quadriceps apparatus.

and thin inner edge; it attaches centrally to the intercondylar tubercles and medially to the capsule. The lateral meniscus attaches to the popliteus and is more mobile than the medial meniscus (and therefore less easily torn). The medial collateral ligament is broad, flat, and attached firmly to both the capsule and the medial meniscus (**252**). The lateral collateral ligament (**254**) is a longer cord-like structure attached to the femur and fibula, independent of the capsule. The two cruciate ligaments (**255, 256**) are named according to their tibial attachments: they are intracapsular, partly covered by synovium, and attached to the condyles in the notch. Knee stability depends on the collateral and cruciate ligaments, the capsule, the patellar ligament and good muscle tone.

The patella keeps the quadriceps tendon 1–2 cm anterior to the femur, increasing its mechanical advantage. The tendency for the patella to undergo lateral translocation (due to the shallower lateral angle of the groove and the lateral pull of the main bulk of quadriceps) is mainly prevented by the pull of the vastus medialis. The vastus medialis, vastus intermedius, and vastus lateralis arise from the femur (**257**) and provide the strong extensor apparatus that stabilises the knee, particularly on weight bearing: the vastus medialis produces the more distal muscle bulge and contracts maximally in the last 10° of extension, taking part in the locking or 'screw home' medial rotation of the femur on the tibia. The rectus femoris (the fourth quadriceps component) arises from the anterior inferior iliac spine and thus acts across two joints.

The main flexors are the hamstrings (the semimembranosus and semitendinosus medially and the biceps femoris laterally, **258**): they are most effective when the hip is flexed. Ancillary flexors are the gracilis, the sartorius and the medial gastrocnemius (medially), and the politeus and the lateral gastrocnemius (laterally). When the knee is flexed ('unlocked') the tibia can rotate on the femur, 40° externally and 30° internally: the lateral hamstrings and tensor fascia lata externally rotate the tibia, and the medial hamstrings and the popliteus internally rotate the tibia.

The knee is involved in most forms of arthropathy; it is also a common site of direct and indirect trauma, which may result in cartilage or ligament damage, enthesopathy, or bursitis.

SYMPTOMS

Pain from the knee (**259**) is predominantly felt anteriorly, often with localisation to the compartment involved (e.g. anteriorly in patellofemoral disease and anteromedially and anterolaterally in medial and lateral compartment problems, respectively). Pain rarely radiates far from the knee: prominent radiation down the tibia normally implies marked subchondral bone collapse or intraosseous hypertension. The front of the knee represents the L2/3 dermatomes (**260, 261**) and pain may be referred to this site from an L3 root lesion or from the hip. Referred pain often differs

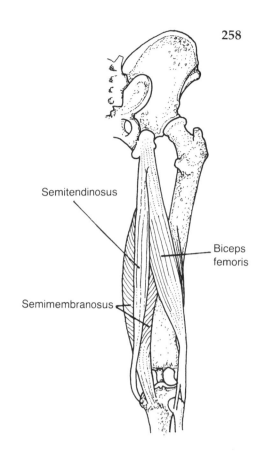

258 Principal knee flexors.

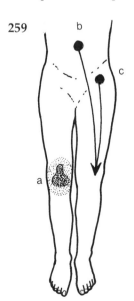

259 Site of pain arising from knee (a), and sites of referred pain to the knee (b, spine; c, hip).

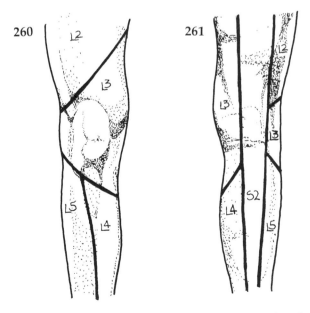

260, 261 Dermatomes around knee: anterior (**260**) and posterior (**261**).

109

from pain originating in the knee in being (1) less clearly demarcated, (2) frequently accompanied by pain and aching above the knee, and (3) exacerbated by different factors. For example, L3 root pain often begins in the buttock, later affecting the front of the thigh and the knee; it is not usually aggravated by walking but may be exacerbated by coughing. The back of the knee represents the S1/2 dermatomes (261). Posterior knee pain alone suggests a complication of arthropathy (e.g. popliteal cyst, posterior tibial subluxation) or an S2 root lesion; other local causes include hamstring or gastrocnemius enthesopathy, lymphadenopathy, and popliteal aneurysm.

'*Locking*' is a sudden, usually transient, painful inability to extend the knee. As a symptom, it is important in suggesting a mechanical derangement, e.g. torn meniscus, 'loose' body, or trapping of a fold of the synovium ('plica' syndrome).

'*Giving way*' describes a feeling of apprehension and loss of confidence in weight bearing on the knee. It predominantly accompanies problems relating to the quadriceps/patellar mechanism or stability. Weakness of the quadriceps, particularly the vastus medialis, or patellofemoral disease, alters vertical 'tracking' of the patella as it moves on the femur and gives rise to this odd feeling of apprehension. Ligamentous instability also alters the mechanics of the knee during weight bearing, so that the patient knows that 'things are not right'.

Patellofemoral abnormalities commonly give rise to two characteristic features in the history:

- Anterior knee pain, which is much worse going up and down (particularly down) stairs or negotiating an incline than walking on the flat. This is because of the maximal stress through that compartment when weight bearing on a flexed knee.
- Progressive anterior knee pain/aching that develops during prolonged sitting with the knee flexed. The patient typically gets up, stretches the legs, and the aching disappears, only to return after 20 min or so of again sitting with knees bent.

INSPECTION

The patient should be inspected while weight bearing and walking and then on a couch at rest. As usual, comparison of one side with the other may help show abnormality associated with unilateral lesions.

Inspection of the standing patient

The patient stands upright and is inspected from in front, the side, and from behind. The main features to observe are deformity and swelling in the posterior popliteal fossa, since these are more apparent when standing than lying.

Deformity

At birth the knee is usually in marked varus: during the toddler and early childhood phases, valgus is common; during adolescence, the knee tends to straighten again. Conditions that cause cartilage loss in both tibiofemoral compartments commonly allow the knee to resume valgus, which is the natural tendency in the majority of individuals.

All deformities other than fixed flexion are best assessed while the patient is standing (262–266): varus and valgus may be noted with the patient lying on the couch, but these are inevitably exaggerated on weight bearing. Principal deformities are:

- *Genu varus* (bow legs). This commonly reflects isolated medial compartment disease (cartilage loss ± subchondral bone collapse) and is the characteristic deformity of uncomplicated osteoarthritis.
- *Genu valgus* (knock knees). This is the usual deformity of arthropathies characterised by synovitis and tricompartmental involvement, leading to cartilage loss throughout the knee.
- *Genu recurvatum*. This is particularly characteristic of generalised hypermobility.
- *Posterior tibial subluxation*. This produces a step-back deformity and is particularly characteristic of arthropathies that affect the developing knee.
- *Fixed flexion*. The knee cannot extend and is always in some degree of flexion. This may complicate a variety of arthropathies, but is particularly common in conditions characterised by synovitis and resolution by fibrosis (e.g. seronegative spondyloarthropathies).

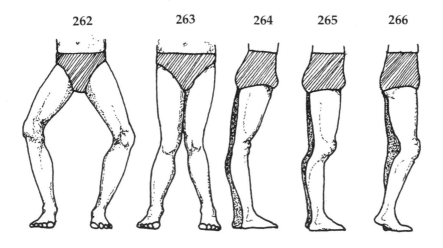

262–266 Knee deformities: (**262**) genu varus; (**263**) genu valgus; (**264**) genu recurvatum; (**265**) posterior tibial subluxation; and (**266**) fixed flexion.

If the patient experiences pain on weight bearing, and a deformity is obvious, manual correction of the deformity (e.g. reducing varus or valgus by pushing from the side) will help suggest whether the pain is predominantly mechanical and, therefore, likely to be helped by correction of the deformity.

Swelling

A popliteal cyst may produce a prominent swelling in the popliteal fossa when the patient is weight bearing and the leg is extended. An abnormally high patella (patella alta) may produce a *'camel sign'* (**267, 268**): because of the high patella (hump 1), the infrapatellar fat pad (hump 2) becomes more prominent. When sitting with knees flexed at 90°, the patellae of such patients may point upwards and be laterally placed (*'frog's eyes'* appearance). Varicose veins should also be noted.

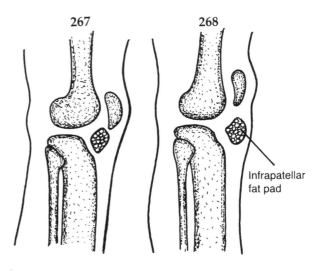

Infrapatellar fat pad

267, 268 Normal patella position (**267**) and two swellings (*'camel sign'*) due to patella alta (**268**).

Inspection of the walking patient

Gait is described in Chapter 2. Look particularly for an antalgic gait, a short step due to fixed flexion, and circumduction of the leg due to fixed extension.

Inspection of the patient lying on a couch

Skin changes

The anterior (extensor) surface of the knee is a common site for psoriasis. Look also for erythema (either localised over a bursa, or more generalised if the knee is involved), scars, or other abnormality.

Swelling

Knee effusion

Fluid collecting in the knee first fills in the medial dimple at the side of the patella and then expands the suprapatellar pouch, giving a horseshoe swelling above and to either side of the patella (**269, 270**).

Bursae/fat pads

Localised swelling in front of the patella suggests prepatellar bursitis (**271**). Localised swelling apparent below the patella, in front of the patellar tendon, suggests a superficial infrapatellar bursitis (**271**); less prominent swelling either side of the tendon suggests deep infrapatellar bursitis or a large infrapatellar fat pad (**272**). A prominent medial fat pad (especially in obese women) may produce a large swelling with ill-defined boundaries above or below the medial joint line; more subtle swelling below the medial joint line may be seen with anserine bursitis.

Muscle

Inspect the quadriceps for wasting (comparison

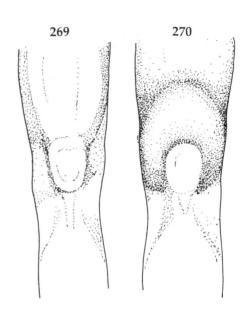

269,270 Normal knee contours (**269**); swelling of knee effusion (**270**).

with the other side is helpful in unilateral lesions). Although all the quadriceps waste uniformly, wasting of the bulky vastus medialis (particularly in a fit young male) may be the most conspicuous. Quadriceps wasting is a difficult sign, particularly in the middle-aged/elderly, and especially in

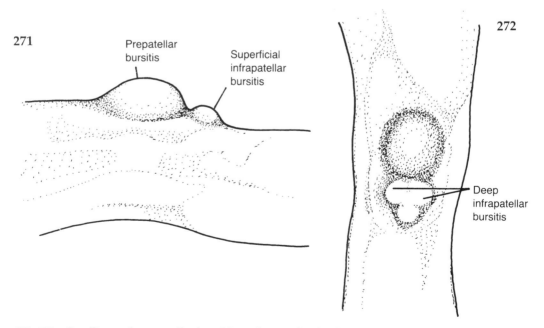

271,272 Swellings of prepatellar bursitis and superficial infrapatellar bursitis (**271**; side view); swelling of deep infrapatellar bursitis (**272**; front view).

women. Some asymmetry of muscle bulk is common and not necessarily abnormal (e.g. it may relate to usage and 'footedness'). Measuring quadriceps (thigh) girth with a tape measure at a fixed point (e.g. 10cm) above the patella on each side is often recommended, but has problems with reproducibility and lack of agreement as to what difference between the sides constitutes abnormality.

Deformity

Fixed flexion is best assessed while the patient is lying and attempts to straighten the legs. Other deformities may also be noted but are usually greater on weight bearing.

Attitude

The way the patient positions the leg and their ease in getting on and off the couch may give an idea of pain severity. The patient will keep returning to a flexed-knee position if there is synovitis or a tense effusion causing intra-articular hypertension.

Palpation

Temperature

Run the back of the hand over the leg anteriorly and down each side, comparing skin temperature above and below the knee to that over the knee. If anything, the knee normally feels cooler than the thigh or shin. Increase in temperature may reflect synovitis (widespread, mainly felt over the whole suprapatellar pouch) or bursitis (localised). If increased warmth is found, be careful this does not relate to varicose veins (often most apparent when standing).

Swelling

Fluid within the joint can be detected by one of three signs.

Bulge sign (273)

This detects a small amount of fluid (and is not necessarily abnormal). Stabilise the patella while gently massaging down either side of the patella, in turn, observing the opposite side around the medial and lateral dimples. A small amount of fluid may flick from one side of the pouch to the other.

Balloon sign

With a moderate/tense effusion, the bulge sign is usually lost and the balloon sign becomes positive (274). Place the palm of one hand over the patella with the fingers and thumb off to the

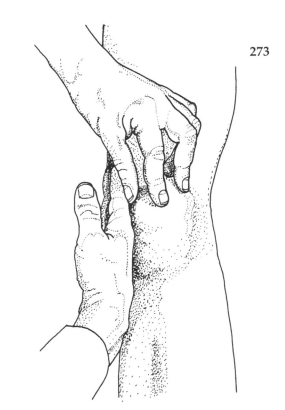

273   Bulge sign.

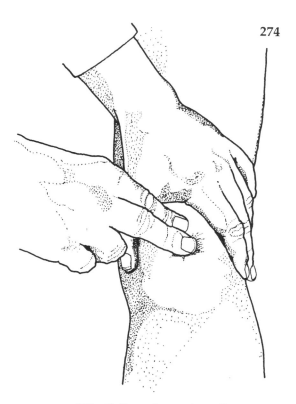

274   Balloon sign and patella tap.

113

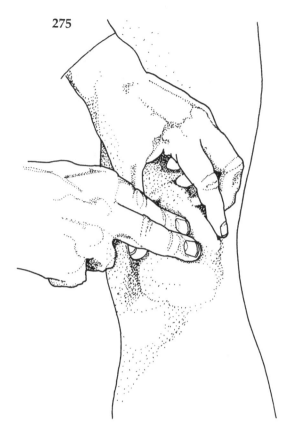

275 Patellofemoral compartment stressing.

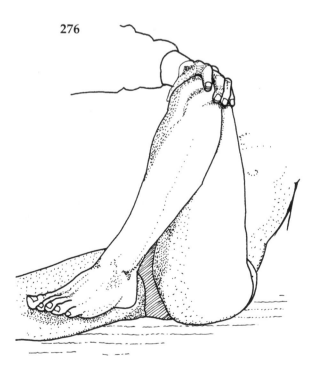

276 Active flexion while feeling for crepitus.

medial and lateral sides; then press firmly down and in with the hand — this automatically encourages fluid to flow down towards the main cavity at the tibiofemoral junction. If pressure is now applied onto the patella or inferior joint region with the other hand 'ballooning' of the first hand is felt. This is the most specific test for fluid in the knee.

Patella tap
While testing for a balloon sign, the patella may be felt to move through the displacing fluid and then 'tap' or 'clonk' onto the femur (**274**). Although common with a large effusion this also occurs with marked retropatellar or anterior femoral fat.

Fluid may be detected in prepatellar or superficial infrapatellar bursitis by placing a finger and thumb either side of the swelling and pressing at its apex for a balloon sign. For deep infrapatellar bursitis, press over the patellar tendon and feel for ballooning to either side. A balloon sign is less commonly present with anserine bursitis.

Patellofemoral compartment
Press the patella back onto the femur with one hand while steadying it with the other (**275**): medial and lateral movement of the patella may then elicit tenderness and give rise to crepitus, felt by both hands. Alternatively, stress the compartment by asking the patient to tighten the quadriceps by pushing the knee backwards into the couch: this pulls the patella onto the femur and may reproduce the pain of which they complain (this procedure produces no hip or other knee compartment movement). Localisation of predominant tenderness to either the medial or lateral facet can be determined by pushing the patella medially and then laterally, in turn, out of its tracking, with the quadriceps well relaxed, while palpating firmly the medial and then lateral facets from each side.

Active assisted and passive movement
The range of active *flexion* is assessed with the examiner's hand draped over all three compartments (palm over the patella, fingers medially, thumb laterally) to detect crepitus at each site (**276**). Observe flexion from the side as the patient attempts to put the heel to the bottom (normally about 115–135°), and enquire concerning pain, particularly in a 'stress pain' pattern (i.e. maximal towards the extremes of limited flexion and extension). Compare active *extension* from the flexed position with passive extension (i.e. lift the heel upwards from the couch): passive extension will correct any 'quadriceps lag' (**277, 278**). Decreased active extension usually results from muscle

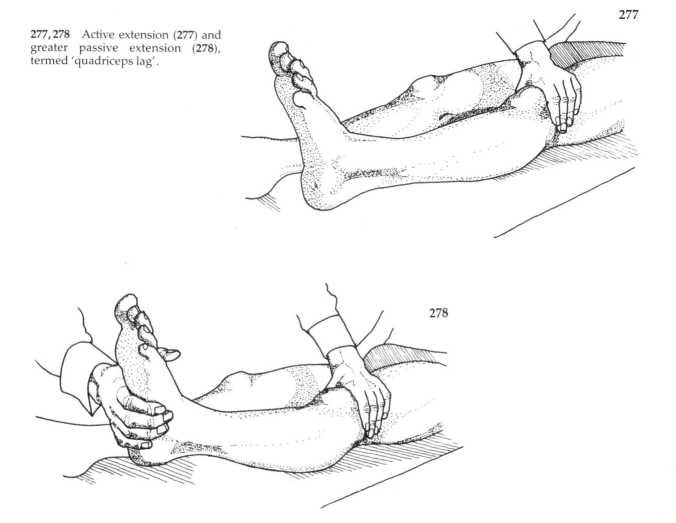

277,278 Active extension (**277**) and greater passive extension (**278**), termed 'quadriceps lag'.

277

278

atrophy (to complete the last 15° of extension a 60% increase in force of quadriceps is required). Extension may also be reduced in joint disease (similar for active and passive), or increased (>10°) in an unstable, damaged knee or in generalised hypermobility.

Tibiofemoral compartments

To identify the joint lines, position the knee in moderate flexion. The *tibial tubercle* is readily found in the midline (**279**), and may be locally tender in Osgood–Schlatter disease. As the palpating finger is taken medially and then proximally from the tubercle the expansion of the tibial plateau is readily identified; as the finger goes higher the anterior joint line is felt as a valley dipping backwards between the tibia (below) and the femoral condyle (above) (**280**). Internal and external rotation of the tibia will open up the lateral and medial joint lines, respectively, and

permit easier identification in difficult cases (e.g. obese subjects). Having found the anterior medial joint line, press firmly just medial to the patellar tendon; then, follow the medial joint line around, pressing firmly all the way. *Tenderness* localised to the anterior joint line is characteristic of medial meniscal injury, whereas more generalised medial joint-line/capsular tenderness suggests arthropathy. Repeat the same procedure for the lateral tibiofemoral joint line; again, localised anterior tenderness suggests meniscal pathology whereas generalised tenderness favours arthropathy.

While palpating both anterior joint lines, the examiner assesses the presence of any soft-tissue swelling. *Synovial thickening* may cause fullness at both anterior joint lines, with a visible convex bulge: if pressed it will give, but then immediately reform as pressure is released. This may be a misleading sign for synovial thickening, since a prominent *infrapatellar fat pad* may appear

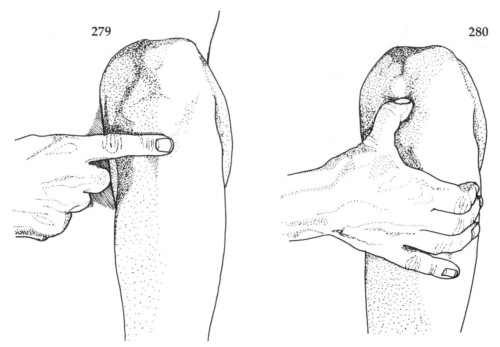

279, 280 Palpation of tibial tubercle (**279**) and anterior joint-line tenderness (**280**; medial tibiofemoral compartment).

identical. *Deep infrapatellar bursitis* is another cause of swelling either side of the patellar tendon; however, it may feel warm, give rise to a balloon sign, and have a more definite medial and lateral boundary. Localised swelling arising laterally, or occasionally medially, from the tibiofemoral joint lines may be due to a meniscal cyst: such a swelling may pop in and out of the joint line as the knee flexes/extends.

Periarticular lesions

Having identified and palpated both tibiofemoral joint lines, palpate for localised sites of periarticular tenderness. There are no visual landmarks and it is best to take a single finger and palpate firmly

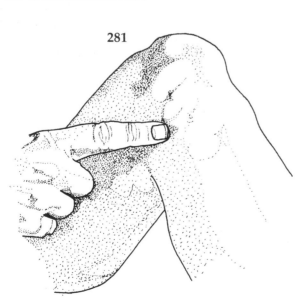

281 Site of tenderness in inferior medial collateral ligament enthesopathy.

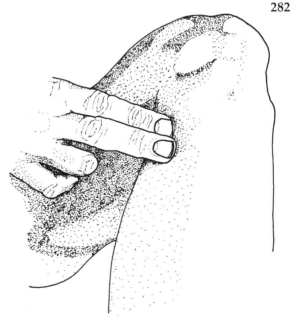

282 Site of tenderness (± swelling) in anserine bursitis.

283 Sites of tenderness in superior medial collateral ligament enthesopathy (localised) and medial fat pad tenderness (diffuse). The examiner's right index finger is overlying the medial joint line.

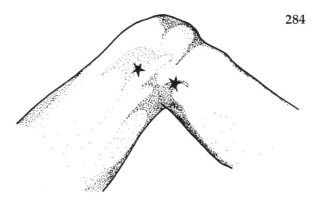

283

over a wide area below, and then above, the joint line on each side. The following lesions are most commonly found.

Inferior medial collateral ligament enthesopathy
This produces localised tenderness inferior to the medial joint line, roughly in the midline of the tibia when observed from the side (this condition is very common, **281**).

Anserine bursitis
This produces a more diffuse area of tenderness inferior to the medial joint line, often overlapping the site of the inferior medial collateral ligament insertion (**282**). It may additionally produce localised swelling, warmth, and, occasionally, a balloon sign. The bursa is named because of the similarity of its contour to that of a webbed goose foot; it lies between the medial collateral ligament and the tendons of sartorius, gracilis, and semitendinosus, close to their insertion (this lesion is common, particularly in middle-aged and elderly subjects).

Superior medial collateral ligament enthesopathy
This produces localised tenderness above the medial joint line, fairly centrally on the femur when observed from the side (**283**).

Medial fat pad syndrome
This produces a wide area of tenderness and 'doughy' swelling superior to, and often overlapping, the medial joint line (this lesion is common, even in non-obese patients). The fat pad is also a common site for tenderness in fibromyalgia.

Inferior lateral collateral ligament enthesopathy
This produces localised tenderness over the fibula head, felt posteriorly on the lateral side (this condition is rare, **284**).

Superior collateral ligament enthesopathy
This causes localised tenderness superior to the lateral joint line, centrally on the femur when observed from the side (**284**). Lateral ligament strains are uncommon sporting injuries that characteristically produce a painful arc under flexion loading at 15–30°.

Iliotibial tract ('band') syndrome
This produces a line of tenderness that extends from the anterolateral tibia, across the joint line, and up the side of the thigh; tenderness is usually maximal over the lateral femoral condyle (**285**). Predominantly a sporting injury, this syndrome also causes a painful arc at about 30°. Pressure over the lateral femoral condyle as the knee is passively moved from full flexion to extension may reproduce pain at about 30° of flexion (Noble compression test).

284

284 Sites of tenderness in inferior and superior lateral collateral ligament enthesopathy.

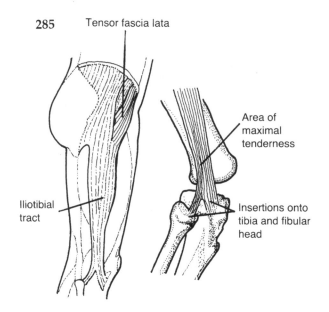

285 Iliotibial tract (band) syndrome.

Tensor fascia lata

Iliotibial tract

Area of maximal tenderness

Insertions onto tibia and fibular head

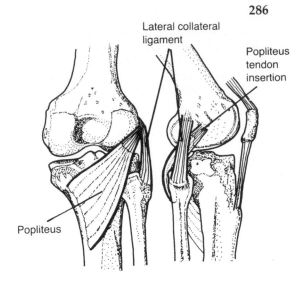

286 Popliteal tendon enthesopathy.

Lateral collateral ligament

Popliteus tendon insertion

Popliteus

Popliteal tendon enthesopathy

This is predominantly a sporting injury that produces localised tenderness on the lateral femoral condyle in a more anterior position than the superior insertion of the collateral ligament (286). It arises, particularly, from running on a cambered, sloped, or uneven track, which strains the popliteus as it attempts to reduce the rotational movement of the tibia on the femur (popliteus problems may be associated with injury to the lateral meniscus, to which it is attached).

The popliteal fossa

This is palpated with the knee in mild-to-moderate flexion: swelling and tenderness are the main features of interest.

Swelling

If a swelling is felt, it may be possible to confirm communication with the joint by massaging its contents back into the main synovial cavity with the knee in flexion. Maintain pressure on the popliteal fossa, extend the knee, then remove both hands: the swelling will not reappear until the patient flexes the knee several times, confirming a valve-like communication between the main cavity and the '*cyst*'. The connection is usually patent only with the knee in mid-flexion, permitting fluid to pass in either direction; as the knee is fully extended or flexed, tendons and other posterior structures close off the valve.

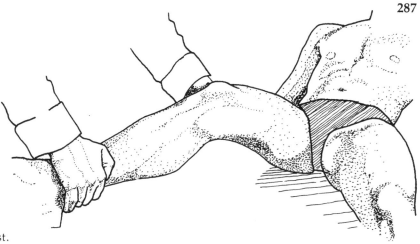

287 Medial ligament stress test.

Tenderness
The medial or lateral hamstring tendons or their insertions, or the medial or lateral insertions of gastrocnemius may be tender to palpation in runners with *hamstring* or *gastrocnemius enthesopathy* (particularly following sprinting or running uphill when these muscles are working at full stretch). Such strains are occasionally accompanied by fine *crepitus* over the tendons.

Stability
Although a large number of tests for instability exist, none is totally specific for a single lesion. The following are standard screening tests for ligament or capsule damage:

Collateral ligaments
Assess stability with the knee 'unlocked' in mild flexion (with the leg straight, the cruciates also prevent lateral movement). Push the femur medially with one hand and the tibia laterally with the other hand (287), looking for excess lateral movement of the tibia (medial ligament instability). As long as sufficient purchase can be achieved to demonstrate this sign the method of holding the leg is immaterial (some examiners place the patient's foot in their armpit and grasp the tibia firmly with both hands to apply greater pressure: 288). In addition to excess lateral movement, also note:

- Opening up of the medial joint line ('*gap sign*').
- *Medial knee pain*, particularly at the inferior insertion of the ligament, suggesting collateral ligament enthesopathy (this manoeuvre is basically a stress test for the medial collateral ligament).

The lateral collateral ligament is similarly tested with the knee in mild flexion, the examiner pushing the tibia medially and the femur laterally.

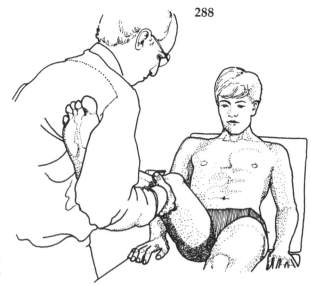

288 Medial ligament stressing using firmer grasp of lower leg.

Again, observe for excess lateral movement, a gap sign, and pain.

Cruciate ligaments
These are examined with the knee flexed to 90° and the hip to 45° (289). Before testing for excess movement:

- Palpate the hamstrings to ensure they are relaxed (otherwise, they may restrict anterior–posterior movement of the tibia and conceal cruciate instability).
- Observe the rounded contour of the knee from the side to ensure the tibia is not starting in a posteriorly subluxed position (*posterior 'sag' sign*) due to posterior cruciate instability.

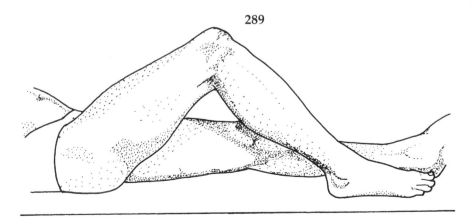

289 Position for cruciate ligament testing.

Having made these checks, test for excess antero-posterior movement of the upper tibia on the femur. Steady the distal tibia with one hand while levering the upper tibia anteriorly and then posteriorly with the other hand (**290**); the patient's weight will hold the femur steady. Some examiners prefer to sit on the patient's foot to steady the lower leg; however, this is unnecessary and may cause pain in those with arthropathy or other painful lesions of the feet. If there is excessive anterior movement (*'anterior drawer' sign*) this may reflect anterior cruciate instability, cartilage loss, or generalised hypermobility. Comparison with the other knee and other tests for hyper-mobility should help interpretation of a positive sign. If the tibia is pushed posteriorly, excess posterior movement implies posterior cruciate instability or, again, cartilage loss or generalised hypermobility.

Lachman's test is a sensitive test for anterior cruciate injury (particularly of the posterolateral fibres). With the knee in mild flexion (<30°) and the patient relaxed, grasp the femur with one hand and the upper shin with the other hand (**291**), and pull the tibia anteriorly to demonstrate excessive movement and a soft 'end feel' (this requires a well-relaxed patient and large examin-ing hands).

If an anterior drawer sign is detected, *Slocum's test* for anterolateral and anteromedial instability may be performed (**292**). With the patient posi-tioned as for the drawer test, sit on the couch and passively rotate the tibia medially 30°, keeping it medially rotated by resting the foot against your buttock. This manoeuvre tightens the lateral cap-sule, giving enough stability then to eliminate the

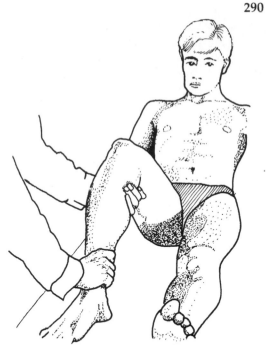

290 Anterior drawer sign.

anterior drawer sign: if the anterior drawer is still positive in this position (most anterior movement occurring on the lateral side) it is likely that the lateral capsule (and/or lateral collateral ligament) is also damaged. Similarly, externally rotate the

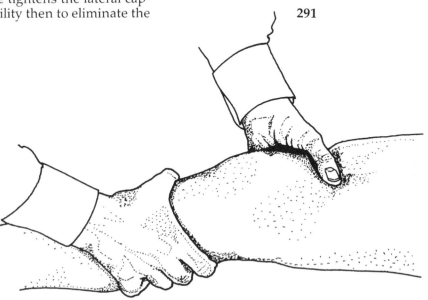

291 Lachman's test.

120

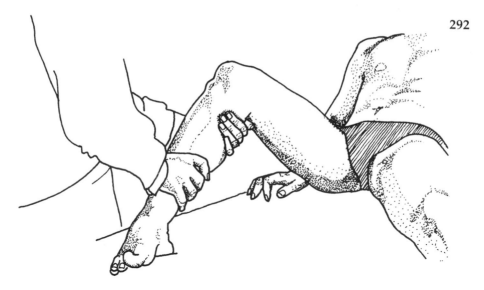

292 Slocum's test.

tibia to tighten the medial capsule: a positive anterior drawer in this position (most movement occurring on the medial side) usually implies that medial capsular fibres (and/or medial collateral ligament) are damaged.

Additional tests for mechanical derangement
If the history (e.g. 'locking') or examination suggests that the problem is primarily mechanical, further tests for mechanical derangement may be of use.

The 'pivot shift' manoeuvre (MacIntosh test)
Another test for anterolateral rotary instability, this manoeuvre is used to demonstrate a dynamic subluxation where the tibia slips laterally and anteriorly on the femur. The patient is positioned supine, with the hip flexed (20°) and relaxed in slight medial rotation, and the knee slightly flexed (5°). The examiner medially rotates the lower tibia with one hand, the other hand pushing the upper tibia anteriorly on the femur while maintaining a valgus stress (**293**). As the knee is then flexed to 30–40° the tibia will suddenly reduce backwards with a 'clunk'. The reduction is due to the iliotibial band moving from an extensor to a flexor function, pulling the tibia back to its normal position. Normally, the knee's centre of rotation changes constantly through its range of motion as a result of the shape of the femoral condyles, ligamentous restraint, and muscle pull. A positive pivot shift test usually suggests damage to the anterior cruciate, the posterolateral capsule, or the lateral collateral ligament.

The mediopatellar plica test
Pain produced by pushing the patella medially with the knee flexed at 30° may be due to a plica squeezed between the femoral condyle and the patella.

The 'apprehension' test
If the patella is carefully pushed laterally with the knee flexed at 30°, the patient may resist, contract the quadriceps, and express insecurity if there is recurrent patellar subluxation or dislocation.

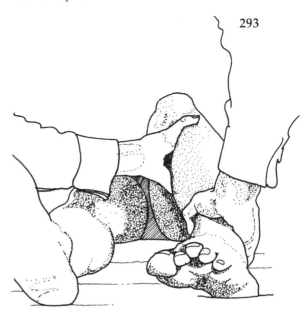

293 Pivot shift test.

SUMMARY OF KNEE EXAMINATION

(1) Inspection of the standing patient
    (a) from in front (particularly for genu valgus, genu varus)
    (b) from the side (particularly for genu recurvatum, posterior tibial subluxation)
    (c) from behind (particularly for popliteal cyst)
(2) Inspection of the walking patient
(3) Inspection of the patient on a couch
    (a) inspection (knee extended) for:
        skin changes
        swelling (effusion, bursae, fat pad)
        quadriceps wasting
        deformity (particularly fixed flexion)
        attitude
    (b) palpation (knee extended) for:
        temperature increase
        swelling (effusion, bursitis)
        patellofemoral tenderness, crepitus
    (c) palpation during flexion (crepitus, restriction, pain)
    (d) passive extension
    (e) palpation (knee flexed)
        tibiofemoral tenderness, swelling
        periarticular tenderness
          collateral ligament enthesopathy
          anserine bursitis
          medial fat pad syndrome
          iliotibial tract syndrome
          popliteal tendon enthesopathy
        popliteal fossa (cyst, tenderness)
    (f) stability of ligaments
        medial/lateral collateral stress tests
        anterior drawer (Slocum's test if positive)
        posterior drawer

9   Ankle and Foot

The lower leg, the ankle, and the foot are well structured for stability in weight bearing and for propulsion during bipedal gait. The large number of bones and their shape permit both flexibility and stability: although movement between individual joints is small, their combined motion permits controlled locomotion over a variety of ground surfaces.

The foot has three functional units:

- The hindfoot (the calcaneus and the talus).
- The midfoot (the five small tarsal bones).
- The forefoot (the metatarsals and the phalanges).

Posteriorly, the bones lie over each other, while in the midfoot and forefoot they lie side by side. This makes the foot higher and narrower at the back, and produces the two (longitudinal and transverse) arches of the foot.

HINDFOOT JOINTS

The *true ankle* (talocrural) joint is a hinged synovial joint between the medial malleolus (tibia), the lateral malleolus (fibula), and the talus (**294, 295**), permitting dorsiflexion and plantar flexion. The fibula aids stability but transmits little weight (the inferior tibiofibular joint is a syndesmosis that permits only a small 'spread' of the ankle mortice during dorsiflexion). Because the trochlea of the talus is wider anteriorly the joint is tighter and more stable in dorsiflexion (as in climbing uphill) than in plantar flexion (descending). The capsule is tightest medially and laterally, where it is bound down by ligaments, but lax in front and behind, being most extensive anteriorly. The enclosed synovial space is usually separate, having no communications.

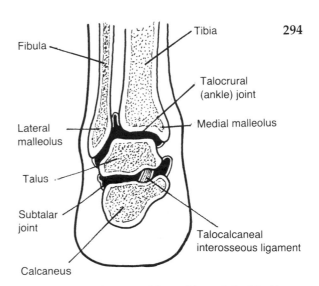

294   Bones and joints of the ankle and the hindfoot.

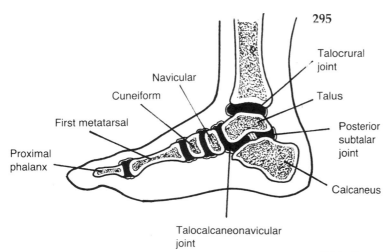

295   Bone and joint arrangement (lateral section).

Stability is maintained by strong collateral ligaments (**296, 297**). The single medial *deltoid ligament* resists eversion of the foot and is very strong (avulsion of the malleolus often occurs before ligament rupture). The lateral ligament is in three bands (the *anterior* and *posterior talofibular ligaments* and the *calcaneofibular ligament*). The anterior talofibular ligament is the first to undergo stress during inversion, and is the most commonly torn. The calcaneofibular ligament may tear, but only after rupture of the anterior talofibular ligament; disruption of both leads to ankle instability. The posterior talofibular ligament is damaged only in severe trauma.

The posterior *subtalar joint* is between the concave undersurface of the talus and the posterior convex facet of the calcaneus (see **295**). The capsule of this deep joint is tight and permits little synovial expansion. Together with the talocalcaneal portion of the talocalcaneonavicular joint, it allows eversion and inversion of the hindfoot.

MIDFOOT JOINTS

The *midtarsal joint* is a functional composite formed mainly by the talocalcaneonavicular and calcaneo-cuboid joints, which permit forefoot eversion and inversion (some forefoot abduction and adduction is also possible). Movement is principally talonavicular but also involves movement between the cuneiform and cuboid bones.

FOREFOOT JOINTS

The *metatarsophalangeal joints* (MTPJs) and proximal and distal *interphalangeal joints* (IPJs) are synovial joints similar to the MCPJs and IPJs of the hand. Each MTPJ capsule is strengthened by a medial and lateral collateral ligament, an extensor tendon dorsally, and a plantar ligament below. MTPJ stability is dependent mainly on the capsule and if capsular function is deranged (e.g. by synovitis) the toes become unstable and follow the pull of the tendons (dorsal subluxation with valgus deformity).

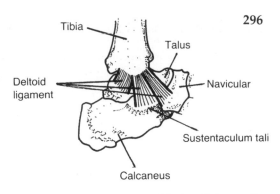

296 Ligaments of the ankle (medial aspect).

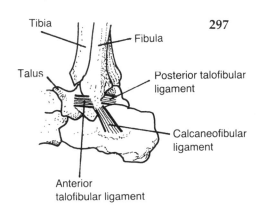

297 Ligaments of the ankle (lateral aspect).

THE ARCH OF THE FOOT

This permits equal weight distribution between the heel prominence (calcaneus) posteriorly and the heads of the lateral four metatarsals and two sesamoid bones of the first metatarsal anteriorly. It provides flexibility and spring for walking and running. The longitudinal arch has a high, flexible medial component and a low, rigid lateral component; the transverse arch is high proximally and low distally. The arch is maintained by the joint capsules and the dorsal and plantar ligaments, and is supported by the long calf muscle tendons (the role of the plantar fascia and small muscles of the sole is uncertain).

TENDONS, BURSAE, AND FASCIA

The *Achilles tendon,* the common insertion of the soleus and the gastrocnemius, attaches to the posterior aspect of the calcaneus and is separated from it by the *retrocalcaneal (pre-Achilles) bursa* (**298**). Other clinically relevant bursae include the *retro-Achilles bursa* (between the skin and the Achilles tendon), the *subcalcaneal bursa* (between the skin and the undersurface of the calcaneus), and adventitious bursae that form over the medial aspect of the first MTPJ ('*bunion*'), and the lateral aspect of the fifth MTPJ ('*bunionette*').

Behind each malleolus run tendons within individual tendon sheaths (**299, 300**):

- Lateral malleolus: the *peroneus longus* and the *peroneus brevis* (eversion), held down by the peroneal retinaculum.
- Medial malleolus: the *tibialis posterior* (inversion) and, more posteriorly, the flexor digitorum longus and the flexor hallucis longus, held down by the flexor retinaculum (forming the *tarsal tunnel* through which also passes the *posterior tibial nerve*).

Anterior and superficial to the ankle are three tendon sheaths held down by the extensor retinaculum (**301**): the medial sheath contains the large tendon of the *tibialis anterior* (the main dorsiflexor of the foot); the central sheath contains the extensor hallucis longus and the extensor digitorum longus; and the lateral sheath contains the peroneus tertius.

The *plantar fascia* arises from the median prominence of the calcaneus. It is tough and thick proximally, but thins as it extends and divides distally before insertion into the bases of the metatarsal heads (see **298**).

The skin on the lateral aspect of the foot, toes, and heel is greatly thickened, and in the subcutaneous connective tissue beneath the metatarsal heads and tips of the toes are *fibro-fatty pads* that act as shock absorbers (**302**). As a result of the concentrated stresses they receive, the foot and ankle are common sites for traumatic articular and periarticular lesions, as well as being target sites for major arthropathies.

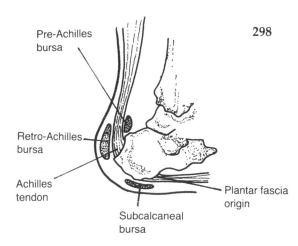

298 Bursae around the ankle.

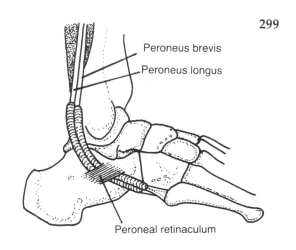

299 Tendons and tendon sheaths around the ankle (lateral).

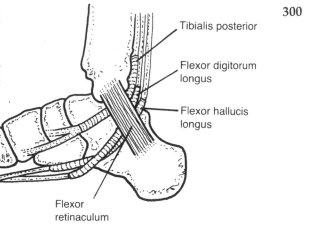

300 Tendons and tendon sheaths around the ankle (medial).

125

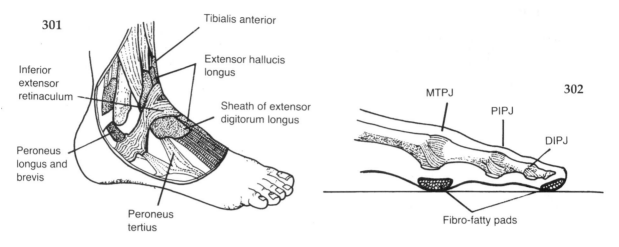

301 Tendons and tendon sheaths around the ankle (anterior)

302 MTPJs and fibro-fatty pads.

SYMPTOMS

Pain arising from articular or periarticular structures is generally well localised and its site and characteristics alone often suggest the cause.

Hindfoot pain

Pain from the ankle joint is felt anteriorly in a broad line joining the two malleoli, and is characteristically worsened by standing or walking. Conversely, pain from the subtalar joint is felt mainly posteriorly between the two malleoli, and is particularly aggravated by walking over uneven surfaces when eversion/inversion is required.

Localised posterior heel pain and tenderness may result from retro-Achilles bursitis, retrocalcaneal bursitis, or Achilles tendinitis or enthesopathy. With Achilles tendon problems, the pain is often exacerbated by standing on tiptoe (without shoes). Pain beneath the heel, which is worsened by prolonged standing or walking, is usually a result of plantar fascia enthesopathy ('plantar fasciitis').

Midfoot pain

Midtarsal joint disease gives pain in the 'bootlace' area, often most marked during late stance and toe-off phases of walking. Loss of the normal arches ('flat foot') may cause pain in the midsole.

Forefoot pain

MTPJ pain is felt below the metatarsal heads (metatarsalgia): it is worsened by standing and walking, and may be described as 'like walking on marbles' if several joints are involved.

Burning pain in the sole and toes suggests a neurogenic cause. Morton's neuroma typically causes sharp intermittent pain between the third and fourth digits, particularly when the metatarsal heads are compressed (as with restrictive shoes). Tarsal tunnel syndrome (posterior tibial nerve entrapment) typically causes burning, tingling, and numbness in the distal sole and toes.

Inflammation of any tendon sheath may cause localised pain that often extends a distance along the line of the sheath and is aggravated by movement of the relevant muscle.

Referred pain

Pain may be referred to the ankle and foot from the spine and, rarely, the hip. Referred pain from nerve-root irritation follows a dermatomal distribution (**303, 304**), may be exacerbated by straining and straight leg raising, and may be accompanied by neurological signs.

EXAMINATION

Inspect both feet and ankles while the patient, undressed to their underwear, stands and then walks. Undertake further inspection and palpation, with the patient resting on a couch. Additional information may be obtained by inspecting the patient's footwear for abnormal moulding and wear patterns of the sole and heel.

Inspection of the standing patient

Compare both sides of the patient, from in front, behind and from the side, looking particularly for the following abnormalities.

Swelling

Ankle synovitis produces diffuse swelling anteriorly (**305**), often filling the small depressions in front of the malleoli. Midtarsal synovitis produces only modest, diffuse puffiness over the dorsum of the midfoot. MTPJ synovitis often causes swelling over the dorsum of the forefoot, obscuring the extensor tendons and causing spreading of the metatarsals and toes. The combination of IPJ synovitis and digital flexor tenosynovitis may produce a 'sausage toe'.

Linear swelling that crosses the ankle is usually a result of extensor tenosynovitis. Peroneal or tibialis posterior tenosynovitis produces linear or diffuse puffiness around the lateral or medial malleolus, respectively.

Swelling around the Achilles tendon may result from tendinitis (producing swelling of the tendon itself), retrocalcaneal bursitis (appearing more as eccentric swelling that fills in either side of the tendon), or retro-Achilles bursitis (more prominent, superficial swelling; **306**). This is also a common site for nodule formation (p. 20), usually appearing as superficial, eccentric swellings over the Achilles tendon and posterior calcaneus.

306 Site of swellings around the Achilles tendon.

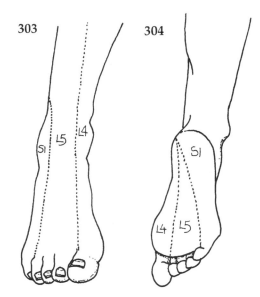

303,304 Dermatomes of the lower leg and the foot: (**303**) dorsal aspect; (**304**) sole.

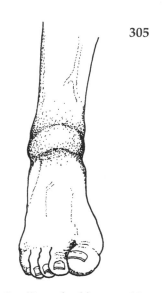

305 Swelling of ankle synovitis.

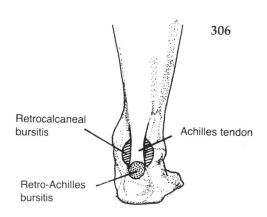

Retrocalcaneal bursitis

Achilles tendon

Retro-Achilles bursitis

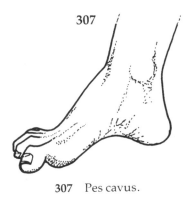

307   Pes cavus.

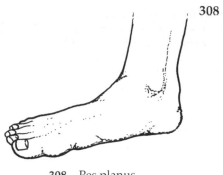

308   Pes planus.

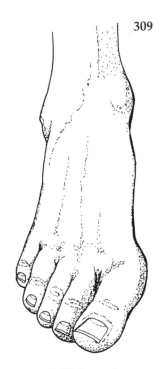

309   Hallux valgus.

Deformity

Ensure that both arches are normal. The longitudinal arch may be increased (*pes cavus*, often a result of neurological disease; **307**) or diminished (*pes planus* or flat foot; **308**). In severe flat foot the displaced talus and navicular cause a prominence in front and just below the medial malleolus.

A large number of joint deformities may be seen. The most common toe abnormality is *hallux valgus* (**309**) in which there is abnormal angulation and rotation of the first MTPJ: associated medial deviation of the metatarsal (metatarsus primus varus) results in a broad forefoot, and a bunion often develops. *Hammertoe deformity* (**310**) results from hyperextension of the MTPJ, with flexion at the proximal interphalangeal joint, or PIPJ (usually the second toe, in association with hallux valgus). The distal interphalangeal joint, or DIPJ, may be straight, flexed or extended and a callus often develops over the prominent PIPJ. *Mallet toe* (**311**) results from flexion deformity at the DIPJ. In *cock-up toe* (**312**) flexion of both IPJs follows extension and often plantar subluxation at the MTPJ (usually due to polyarthritis). The fibro-fatty pad moves distally, and secondary callus may form below the exposed metatarsal head and over the flexed PIPJ.

Ankle and subtalar deformities are best seen from behind. Calcaneovalgus (*eversion*) is most common (**313, 314**), usually reflecting damage to both the subtalar and ankle joint: calcaneovarus (*inversion*) only occasionally occurs. Fixed plantar flexion (*talipes equinus*) usually results from spastic paresis. Congenital clubfoot (talipes) may associate with plantar flexion of the ankle (talipes equinus) or dorsiflexion (*talipes calcaneus*). Midfoot deformity may coexist; for example, *talipes equinovarus* or *talipes cancaneovalgus*.

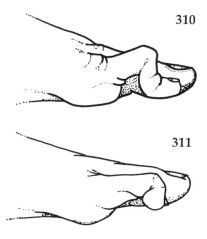

310,311   Toe deformities: (**310**) hammertoe; (**311**) mallet toe.

Skin and nail changes

Relevant observations may include loss of hair over the distal limbs (vascular insufficiency, neuropathy), vasomotor changes and discoloration (Raynaud's disease, vascular disease, cryoglobulinaemia), ulceration (gravitational, vasculitis), and psoriatic plaques. As with the fingers (pp. 21, 38), inspect the nails for pitting and dystrophy (psoriasis, chronic Reiter's syndrome), vasculitic lesions, and clubbing. Peculiar to toenails, usually the hallux, is onychogryphosis (gross distortion and hypertrophy).

Inspection of the walking patient

Gait is described in Chapter 2. Pain in any part of the foot or ankle may give an *antalgic gait*. Other typical abnormalities may suggest the site of involvement.

Hindfoot problem

If ankle movement is reduced, the leg may be externally rotated and slightly abducted, giving a 'toe-out' gait with outward displacement of the forefoot, the patient attempting to walk by rolling the foot from the lateral to the medial side. If severe, this results in loss of the longitudinal arch so the patient walks on the medial aspect of the foot. If the heel is painful, heel strike is avoided, the step being shortened and the forefoot striking first. With Achilles tendon problems, push off is guarded or avoided, the step again being shortened.

Midfoot problem

The foot is often held inverted and push off is from the lateral side.

Forefoot problem

To avoid weight bearing on the forefoot, the heel does not rise in late stance and there is diminished push off. The trunk, hip, and knee flex to maintain forward motion, and swing phase on the normal side shortens, resulting in 'bobbing' during late stance on the painful side. Involvement of both forefeet combines to give a forward-leaning, short-stepped, shuffling gait.

Examination of the recumbent patient

With the patient relaxed on the couch, complete inspection by examining the soles; then undertake palpation and examination of a range of movements.

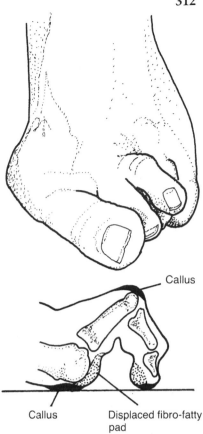

312

312 Cock-up toe deformity with hallux valgus (due to polyarthritis).

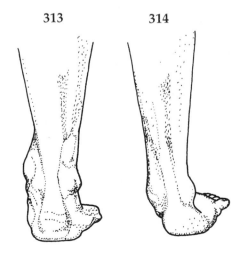

313   **314**

313,314 Normal hindfoot (**313**); hindfoot eversion deformity (**314**).

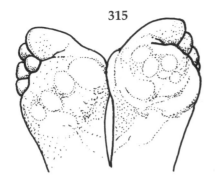

315

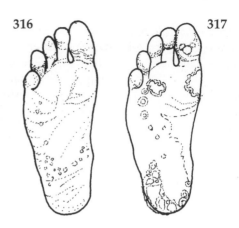

316   317

315 Bursae beneath subluxed MTPJs.

316,317 Keratoderma blennorrhagica: (**316**) early mild; (**317**) established, severe.

Examination of the soles and the interdigital clefts

Callosities and inflamed *adventitious bursae* are particularly common under subluxed MTPJs (**315**). They appear to merge into the surrounding skin and may be tender to direct pressure. Complications that may be present (particularly in rheumatoid disease) include vasculitic lesions, broken skin with discharge, and secondary infection. *Verrucae* are tender to direct and, particularly, laterally applied pressure, and show clear demarcation from surrounding skin. Pustular *psoriatic lesions* and *keratoderma blennorrhagica* appear identical (**316, 317**), and *plantar erythema* is occasionally observed, as on the palms. Part and inspect the interdigital clefts: macerated skin with fissuring is typical of *tinea pedis* (athlete's foot) — common in patients with toe deformities and abnormal skin clefts.

Palpation

Increased warmth

Pass the back of the hand down the dorsum of the foot to feel for increased warmth overlying the ankle, midtarsal joints, or the MTPJs.

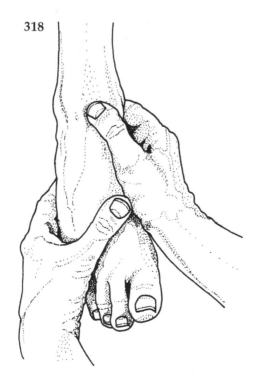

318

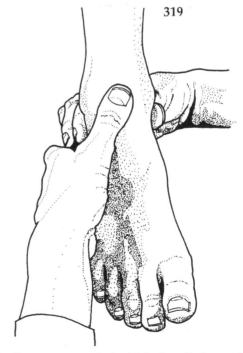

319

318   Palpation of the anterior joint line of the ankle.

319   Pressure posteriorly (right hand), increasing anterior swelling (palpable with left hand).

130

Joint tenderness, swelling, and movement
Work through each joint group looking for:

- Joint-line tenderness.
- Soft-tissue swelling arising from the joint.
- Restriction of passive movement.
- Pain (especially stress pattern) during movement.

Ankle. Identify the anterior joint line by palpating with one or both thumbs while gently dorsiflexing and plantarflexing the ankle (**318**). Note any crepitus during this movement. Having identified the joint line, press firmly for tenderness, and feel for swelling. Synovitis and effusion are most prominent here because of the slack, extensive anterior capsule: such intracapsular swelling becomes more obvious during passive dorsiflexion of the ankle and if pressure is applied over the posterior capsule by a cupped hand pressing beneath and behind both malleoli (**319**).
Movement: with the knee moderately flexed and gastrocnemius relaxed, support the lower leg with one hand, holding the foot firmly with the other hand, and passively move the ankle into dorsiflexion (about 20°; **320**) and plantar flexion (about 45°; **321**).

Subtalar joint. This joint is too deep for palpation and swelling cannot be seen.
Movement: stabilise the distal leg with one hand and, grasping the heel with the other hand, move the foot into inversion (about 30°; **322**) and eversion (about 20°; **323**).

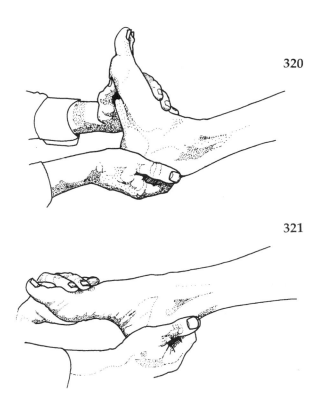

320,321 Ankle dorsiflexion (**320**) and plantar flexion (**321**).

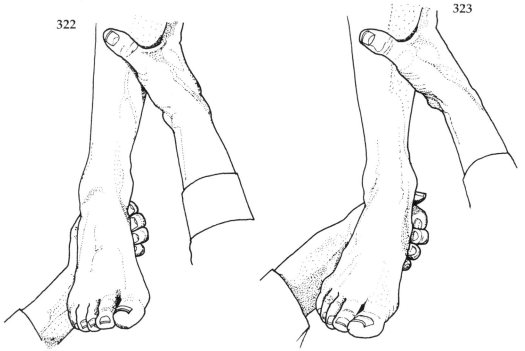

322,323 Subtalar joint movement: inversion (**322**) and eversion (**323**).

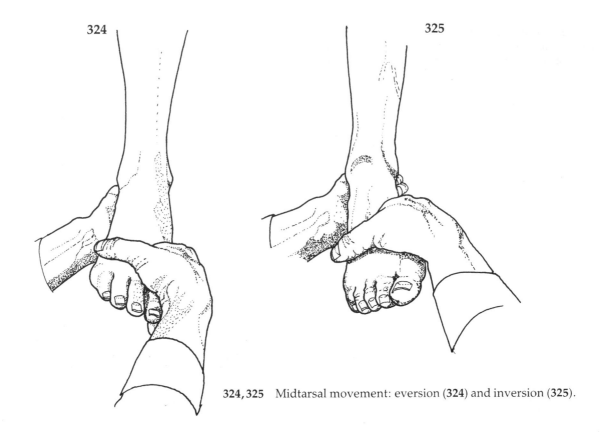

324, 325 Midtarsal movement: eversion (**324**) and inversion (**325**).

Midtarsal joints. Feel for tenderness and soft-tissue swelling over the dorsum of the midfoot. The muscle belly of the extensor digitorum brevis on the lateral aspect of the dorsum may simulate synovial thickening of the ankle or midtarsal joint: it is distinguished by active toe extension, which shortens, bunches up, and hardens the muscle. Bony swelling over the dorsum occurs with talonavicular osteoarthritis, and with prominence of the talus in pes cavus (sometimes with overlying callus formation).

Movement: stabilise the calcaneus in one hand and, holding the forefoot in the other hand, rotate the foot along its long axis into eversion (about 40°; **324**) and inversion (about 30°; **325**).

MTPJs. MTPJ tenderness is elicited by squeezing the forefoot laterally across the metatarsal heads (**326**). If tenderness is elicited the responsible joints are located by palpating each MTPJ in turn, squeezing between both thumbs (on the postero-lateral aspect) and forefingers (plantar aspect; **327**). Synovitis of MTPJs produces dorsal swelling that comes proximally, filling in the spaces between the metatarsal heads. Tenderness of a single metatarsal head may indicate a stress fracture (most commonly the second or third — 'March fracture'). Sharply localised tenderness

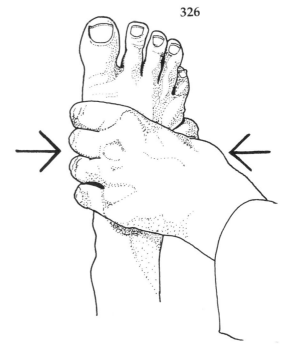

326 Metatarsal squeeze.

between the third and fourth (less commonly second and third) metatarsal heads is characteristic of Morton's interdigital neuroma: altered sensation may be detected on the lateral and medial aspects of the third and fourth toes, respectively, and rarely a large neuroma may be felt.

Movement: test each MTPJ by supporting the metatarsal head between the finger and thumb, and moving the proximal phalanx into extension and flexion (**328**). The first MTPJ has about 80°

extension and 35° flexion; the other MTPJs have about 40° of extension and flexion.

IPJs. Palpate for tenderness of symptomatic or abnormal IPJs by squeezing the posterolateral aspects of each IPJ between the finger and thumb (**329**). Swelling of synovitis is most prominent on the posterolateral and lateral aspects.

Movement: IPJs are tested by fixing the more proximal and moving the more distal phalanx (**330**). PIPJs flex to about 50° and DIPJs to about 40°, with varying extension up to 30°.

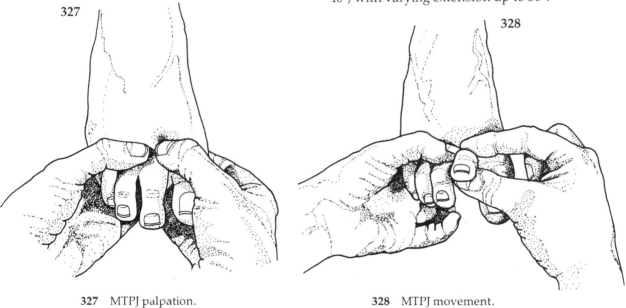

327 MTPJ palpation.

328 MTPJ movement.

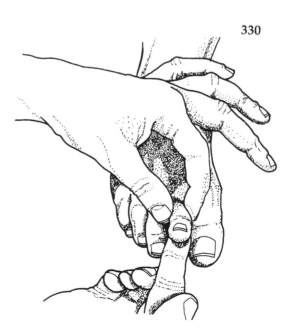

329 Palpation of IPJ.

330 IPJ movement.

Periarticular structures

Palpate behind and under each malleolus for soft-tissue swelling, tenderness, and warmth relating to tendon sheaths. Crepitus may be detected, and pain reproduced, by palpating the relevant tendon sheath with one hand (**331**) while the other hand passively moves the forefoot into eversion (stressing tendons around the medial malleolus) or inversion (stressing the peroneals around the lateral malleolus).

Tenosynovitis overlying the anterior aspect of the ankle is distinguished from ankle synovitis by:

- Its more superficial, linear configuration.
- Tenderness extending well beyond the joint line.
- Pain produced by the appropriate resisted active movement (dorsiflexion of the foot, extension of the hallux and toes).

Plantar fasciitis is confirmed by reproducing pain by firm pressure over the midpoint of the heel (**332**).

Examination of the posterior heel and Achilles is best undertaken with the patient lying prone, with the feet extending beyond the end of the couch. Palpate (between the forefinger and thumb) for tenderness and swelling of:

- The Achilles tendon (Achilles tendinitis, partial rupture).
- The tissues anterior and lateral to the tendon (pre-Achilles bursitis).
- The tendon insertion site into the calcaneus (retro-Achilles bursitis or Achilles enthesopathy).

Then, test for resisted active plantar flexion by asking the patient to push their foot down against your hand (**333**). This may reproduce pain in Achilles tendinitis, enthesopathy, or partial rupture, but not bursitis. In partial rupture, a defect in the tendon, which becomes more noticeable during resisted plantar flexion, may be palpable.

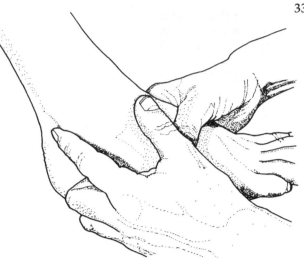

331 Palpation for peroneal tendon sheath crepitus.

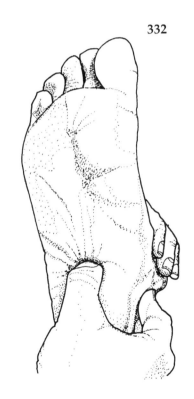

332 Tenderness due to plantar fasciitis.

With complete rupture of the tendon, resisted active movement is absent, and firm squeezing of the relaxed gastrocnemius (shortening it) will not produce any passive plantar flexion. Old (healed) partial rupture may leave a palpable nodule in the tendon.

Palpate other nodules (due to generalised disease) to determine attachment to the skin or to underlying structures.

Additional tests for stability

Anterior stability

The anterior drawer sign tests the integrity of the anterior talofibular ligament. With the patient sitting, push back on the lower tibia with one hand while pulling the calcaneus and talus anteriorly with the other hand (**334**). Any movement of the foot relative to the tibia indicates instability.

Lateral instability

This results from anterior talofibular and calcaneofibular ligament damage. Hold the calcaneus in both hands and palpate beneath the lateral malleolus with one thumb (**335**). Slowly invert the heel, looking for excess movement and development of a palpable 'gap' beneath the laterally placed thumb. For deltoid ligament insufficiency (an uncommon condition), evert the calcaneus and feel for a gap on the medial side.

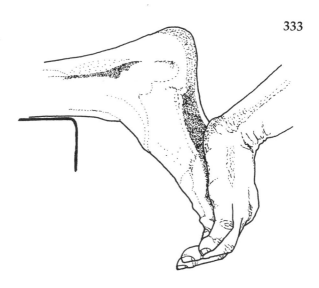

333 Resisted active plantar flexion.

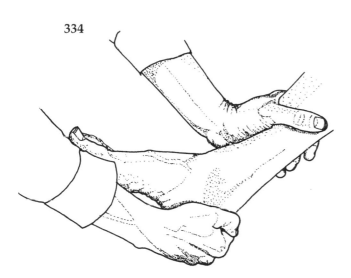

334 Test for anterior instability.

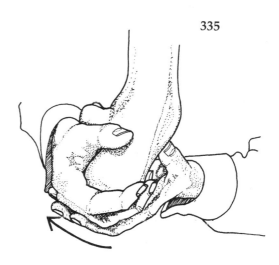

335 Test for lateral instability.

SUMMARY OF FOOT EXAMINATION

(1) Inspection of the standing patient
    (a) swelling (synovitis, tenosynovitis, tendinitis, bursitis, nodules)
    (b) deformity (arches, joints)
    (c) skin, nails
(2) Inspection of the walking patient
(3) Examination of the recumbent patient
    (a) inspection of soles, interdigital clefts
    (b) palpation (warmth, swelling, tenderness) and movement (restriction, pain, crepitus) of joints:
        ankle (dorsiflexion/plantar flexion)
        subtalar (inversion/eversion of calcaneus)
        midtarsal (inversion/eversion of midfoot)
        MTPJs (flexion/extension)
        IPJs (flexion/extension)
    (c) palpation (warmth, swelling, tenderness) with or without movement (pain, crepitus) of periarticular structures:
        tenosynovitis (extensors, peroneals, tibialis posterior)
        plantar fascia insertion
        Achilles tendon and insertion (patient prone)
        pre-Achilles, retro-Achilles bursitis (patient prone)
    (d) tests for stability (anterior, lateral)

10 Temporomandibular Joint

The mandible articulates as a single unit with the skull at three sites: the two temporomandibular joints (TMJs) and the teeth (the 'trijoint complex'). The TMJs are among the most frequently used joints in the body, the jaw opening and closing about 2000 times each day as we chew, suck, swallow, talk, kiss, yawn, snore, etc.

Each TMJ has fibro (not hyaline) articular cartilage, and a fibrocartilage disc completely divides the cavity into two synovial compartments (336). The upper compartment functions as a *sliding* joint (permitting anteroposterior and some lateral movement of the mandible); the lower compartment acts as a *hinge*. On opening the mouth the condylar heads rotate; then the condyles and discs both slide forward on the temporal articulations (337–339). The joint capsule is lax but condensed laterally as the temporomandibular ligament; the stylomandibular and sphenomandibular ligaments are further restraints that keep the condyle, disc, and temporal bones opposed. In general, however, the loose capsule and non-restraining bony configuration allow the condylar position to be easily influenced by occlusal, muscular, and postural factors, and by trauma.

The lateral pterygoids are the prime openers of the mouth and pull each condyle and disc forwards: acting together they protrude the jaw; acting individually they laterally deviate it. The masseter, the temporalis, and the internal pterygoids are prime closers; the temporalis is the prime retractor.

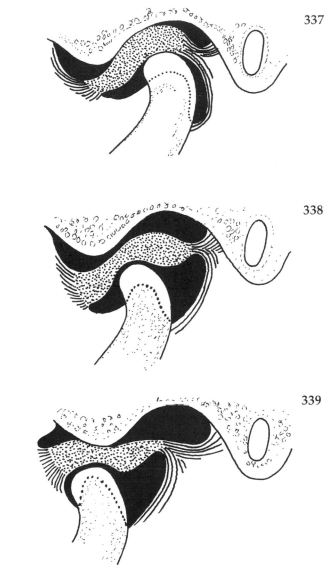

337

338

339

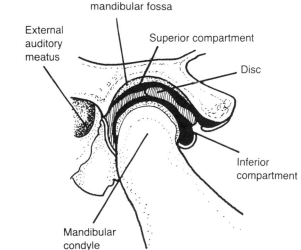

336

External auditory meatus

Fibrocartilage of mandibular fossa

Superior compartment

Disc

Inferior compartment

Mandibular condyle

Mandibular condyle

336 Outline of basic temporomandibular joint anatomy.

337–339 Normal TMJ opening: (**337**) the mouth closed; (**338**) the mouth opening — the condyle rotates and moves anteriorly with the disc; (**339**) the mouth fully open.

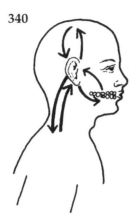

340 Referred pain patterns to and from the TMJ.

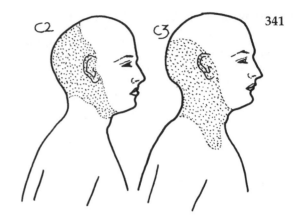

341 Dermatomes around the TMJ.

Pain from a TMJ may be felt locally, but is most commonly referred to the mandible, the teeth, the side of the head, or the neck (**340**). Less commonly, pain from the teeth or neck may be referred to the TMJ area, which approximates to the junction of the C2 and C3 dermatomes (**341**).

The TMJs and teeth depend on each other for normal development and function. If TMJ pain is suspected, specific enquiry should include:

- *Pain* on opening or closing the mouth, on chewing, yawning, or talking. (If so, where is it felt?)
- *Locking* of the jaw (locking in the closed position is usually due to disc problems, locking in the open position to subluxation).

- '*Clicking*' of the jaw (often due to partial sub-luxation or damage to the disc, lateral pterygoid dysfunction, or to occlusal imbalance).
- Previous or current problems with *teeth* (caries, malocclusion, extraction, dentures).
- Occurrence of '*bruxism*' (forced clenching/grinding of the teeth, especially at night, which may cause TMJ pain).
- *Ear* problems (hearing loss, blocking of the ears, earache, or dizziness may denote ear, neck, or TMJ problems).

EXAMINATION

Inspection at rest

Observe and compare the location of each TMJ just anterior to the external auditory meatus. **Swelling** from the joint has to be marked before it can be seen as a rounded bulge overlying this site. **Erythema** (often accompanied by more wide-spread soft-tissue swelling) suggests sepsis or crystal synovitis. Ask the patient to bare teeth and observe for any **overbite, crossbite,** or **lateral deviation** of the jaw. TMJ disease during growth may lead to general hypoplasia of the jaw and a receding chin ('**micrognathia**', **342**).

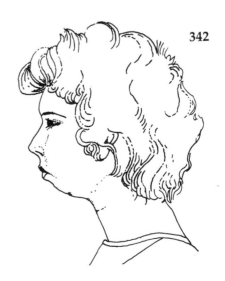

342 Micrognathia.

Inspection during movement

Each movement should show a smooth, unbroken rhythm and be painfree. Ask the patient to:

- *Open the mouth wide* (**343**). The mouth should open and close in a vertical line. Hypomobility of one TMJ causes jerky movement, with regular deviation of the jaw to that side on opening, and deviation away from that side on closing. Variable side-to-side jerkiness on opening or closing more often relates to muscle imbalance (e.g. following neck hyperextension injury). The jaw normally opens about 3–6 cm, sufficient to accommodate two or three flexed fingers (**343**).

- *Protrude the jaw forwards* (**344**). The bottom teeth should easily be placed in front of the top teeth and there should be no lateral deviation.
- *Move the jaw from side to side* (**345**). With the jaw protruded, this permits greater lateral movement — normally about 1–2 cm. TMJ disease may cause earlier and greater loss of lateral movement than of vertical movement.

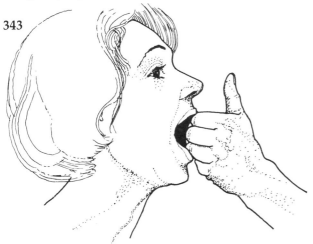

343 Mouth opening (normal from the front, accommodation of three flexed fingers held vertically).

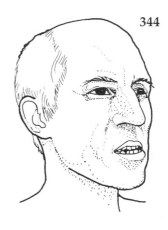

344 Jaw protrusion.

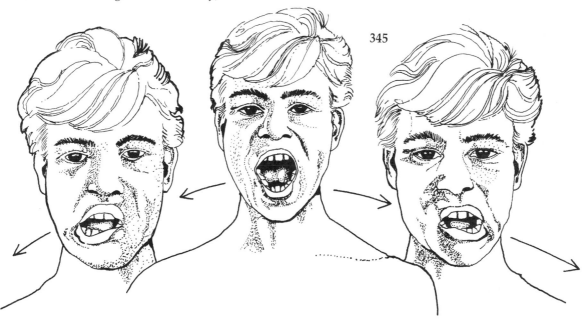

345 Lateral jaw movements.

Palpation

Feel for increased **warmth** with the back of the hand over the region just anterior to the external meatus. Place the index fingers of each hand over the same TMJ areas and ask the patient to open and close the mouth: the palpating fingers will be felt to drop into a depression overlying the joint as the condyles move forward. Fluid/soft-tissue **swelling** prevents easy palpation of this depression and may, additionally, give rise to a balloon sign (fluctuance). **Crepitus** or **clicking** may be palpable during movement and comparison of palpable movements on the two sides permits detection of varying degrees of subluxation. Pressure over this area may elicit **tenderness**.

Palpation of the posterior aspect of the TMJ is accomplished by placing the tips of each little finger into each external meatus (fingernails pointing posteriorly) and pressing anteriorly as the patient opens and closes the mouth (**346**). If synovitis is present, tenderness on mouth closure is more readily appreciated at this site than on palpation over the lateral aspect.

Resisted active (isometric) movement is difficult to perform but useful in differentiating muscle dysfunction from TMJ disease. The jaw should be in the resting (just open) position. Test:

- *Opening* (prime movers = the lateral pterygoids), by asking the patient to resist an increasing closing force applied by the examiner's hand under their chin (with their head supported by the other hand to prevent neck extension: **347**).
- *Closing* (the masseter, the temporalis, and the medial pterygoids), by asking the patient to resist an increasing opening force applied by the examiner's hand to the biting surfaces of their lower anterior teeth (or chin, if diseased/absent teeth), while supporting their forehead with the other hand to prevent neck flexion (**348**).

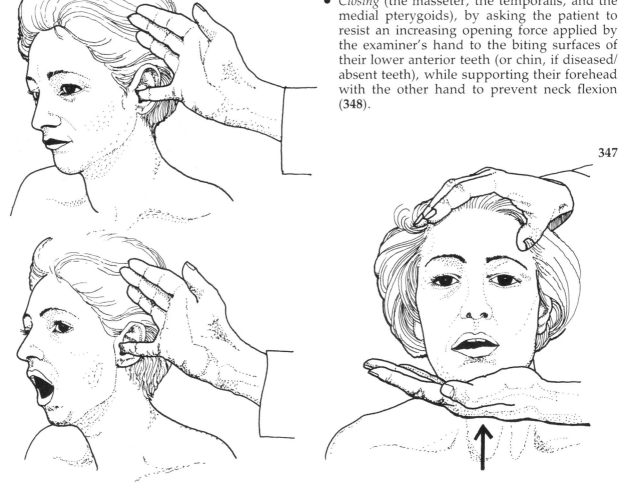

346 Palpation of the posterior aspect of the TMJ as the patient opens and closes the mouth.

347 Resisted isometric mouth opening: the examiner prevents the patient opening her mouth.

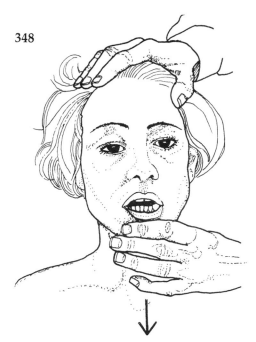

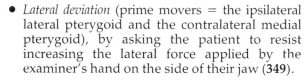

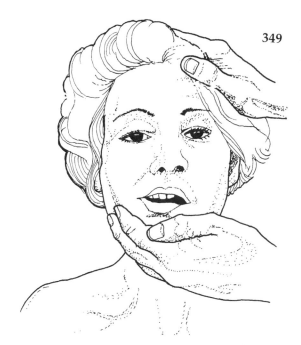

348 Resisted isometric mouth closure: the examiner prevents the patient closing her mouth.

349 Resisted isometric lateral deviation: the examiner prevents the patient pushing her jaw laterally (to her right).

- *Lateral deviation* (prime movers = the ipsilateral lateral pterygoid and the contralateral medial pterygoid), by asking the patient to resist increasing the lateral force applied by the examiner's hand on the side of their jaw (**349**).

In addition, the lateral pterygoids may be palpated by placing a gloved finger between the cheek and the upper gum and pushing backwards beyond the last molar against the neck of the mandible.

As the patient opens their mouth the lateral pterygoid is felt to tighten against the examiner's fingertip. If the muscle has been traumatised or is in spasm, pain or tenderness may be elicited.

Inspection and palpation of teeth and gums (e.g. for caries, gingivitis, loose/malfitting dentures) should also be undertaken if warranted. Palpate the gums and teeth with a gloved finger, looking for localised tenderness and easy gum bleeding.

SUMMARY OF TMJ EXAMINATION

(1) Inspection at rest (swelling, erythema, micrognathia)
(2) Inspection of bared teeth (overbite, crossbite, lateral deviation)
(3) Inspection during movement
      open mouth wide
      protrude jaw forwards
      move jaw from side to side
(4) Palpation
      warmth
      swelling
      tenderness (anterior and posterior compartments)
      crepitus/clicking during movement
(5) Resisted active movements
      jaw opening
      jaw closing
      lateral deviation
(6) Inspection and palpation inside mouth
      (lateral pterygoids, teeth, gums)

INDEX